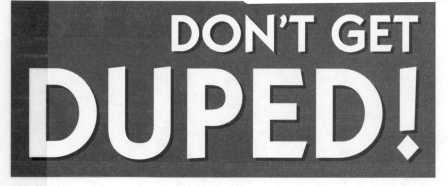

DON'T GET DUPED!

A
CONSUMER'S
GUIDE TO
HEALTH
AND FITNESS

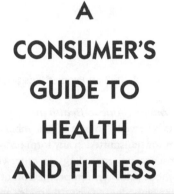

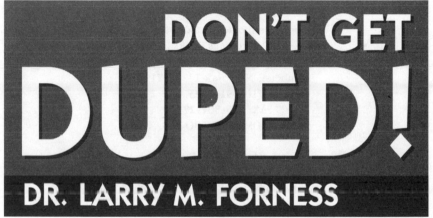

DON'T GET
DUPED!

DR. LARRY M. FORNESS

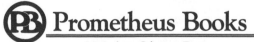 Prometheus Books

59 John Glenn Drive
Amherst, New York 14228-2197

Published 2002 by Prometheus Books

Inquiries should be addressed to
Prometheus Books
59 John Glenn Drive
Amherst, New York 14228-2197
VOICE: 716-691-0133, ext. 207
FAX: 716-564-2711
WWW.PROMETHEUSBOOKS.COM

06 05 04 03 02   5 4 3 2 1

Library of Congress Cataloging-in-Publication Data

Forness, Larry M., 1943–
    Don't get duped! : a consumer's guide to health and fitness / Larry Forness.
        p. cm.
    Includes bibliographical references and index.
    ISBN 1-57392-922-0 (pbk. : alk. paper)
    1. Health. 2. Physical fitness. 3. Consumer education. I. Title.

RA776 .F697 2001
613.7—dc21   2001048275

Printed in the United States of America on acid-free paper

TOP GUN

You came into my life 15 August 1988.
You died in my arms 30 August 1998.
No one ever had any living thing that was so full of love,
trust, friendship, and companionship.

You were my dog.
My Silent Sentinel.

You are my Eternal Companion.

I will love you forever.

CONTENTS

ACKNOWLEDGMENTS

The author gratefully acknowledges the best friend he ever had in his life, known to all that knew him as "Top Gun." He was the inspiration for not only this book, but others, and served as a model for love, loyalty, companionship, and truth. He gave me everything he had every day of his life. He was my dog. He died in my arms of a heart attack on the night of 30 August 1998. I will see you again, my friend, and then we will be together for all eternity. We are eternal companions.

Thanks are due to my wonderful assistant, Anne Parsons, who is responsible for many of the tables in, and editing of, this book. I know her work is often unnoticed by others, but she is a joy to work with and a true lady.

I must offer my sincere thanks to my agents, Barbara Harris and Norman Rudenberg, for their editorial advice, friendship, patience, and professional conduct.

Special gratitude is extended to editor-in-chief Steven L. Mitchell and senior editor Mary A. Read of Prometheus Books for their peerless guidance and demeanor.

Last, thank you, Lord, for giving me the brains (such as they are) and talent in my chosen profession. I could do nothing without you.

DISCLAIMER

Nothing in this book is intended as medical advice by the author.

Nothing in this book should be construed as medical advice by any reader.

The reader is always directed, first and foremost, to his or her own personal physician for specific medical advice and/or treatment, as well as before beginning any exercise or weight-loss program.

The author assumes no responsibility for the use or misuse of any information contained herein by anyone for any purpose.

INTRODUCTION

The information in this book could save you money—perhaps a *lot* of money. It could certainly save you considerable frustration, embarrassment, and disappointment. *It could even save your life.*

What is contained in these pages may anger and shock you. It might well make you laugh. It will entertain, educate, and strengthen you. It will definitely change the way you look at health and fitness ads.

You will be given specific examples of the incredibly powerful subtleties that prey on your mind and your pocketbook. You're going up against some real professionals when it comes to misinformation and deceptive claims. You'll read and see exactly how they do it to you.

I have a confession to make. I've been suckered for forty years by misleading claims and incorrect information by those who manufacture and promote vitamins, minerals, ergogenic supplements, herbs, fitness equipment, fitness apparel, and "alternative" health care. And I'm supposed to be an expert on these items!

It all started in 1959 when my parents bought me my first set of free weights for my sixteenth birthday. I was ready to try out for football and, at six feet, two inches tall and tipping the scales at 140 pounds, I needed to put on some weight before I got annihilated on the playing field.

The weights were purchased from a company run by a now-famous manufacturer of bodybuilding equipment. With the weights came a page that said that if you wanted "personal advice" on building up a certain part of your body to send two dollars in cash to another guy—a bodybuilder—with your question, and he'd respond.

I sent away the question with the two dollars.

Got no answer. I did it again.

Got no answer. Did it a third time.

Got no answer.

Finally, I dialed Information, got the company's phone number, called them, and demanded my money back. The response I got on the phone was "Go to hell, kid," and the guy hung up on me! That planted the seed for this book. And I hope it truly is a case of "What goes around, comes around."

That six dollars wasn't a load of money, but the total amount of money wasted on the practices and products debunked in this book amount to many billions of dollars per year.

Collectively, the chapters in this book will give you fact, not fluff, so you can stop wasting your hard-earned money on false claims. I will also show you what you need to know to truly be "an informed consumer"—someone who doesn't get duped.

Specifically, chapter 1, "How and Why You Get Duped: The Head Game," will illustrate in detail exactly how the health and fitness industry gets inside your head to separate you from your money. It might be subtitled "The Psychology of Deception." You'll see some of the many ways the industry advertises its products to draw you in.

Chapter 2, "The Scientific Method: How to Prove What *Is* the Truth," explains how something is "scientifically proven." There is only one legitimate way to prove the validity of a statement or claim made in the industry. Though the scientific method can be technical, I describe it in plain and simple terms.

Chapter 3, "How *You* Can Measure the Claims *and* the Results: The Quantitative versus the Qualitative," shows how you can actually measure the claims and the results. Claims such as "more energy," "increased fitness level," "improve strength," "shed pounds," and the like are either false or misleading; thus, *all are useless*. They are *qualitative* statements. You need and deserve the *quantitative* amounts; that is, *how much and how fast*? I'll show you how to get this information.

Chapters 4 through 9 discuss the many items you can buy. I'll tell you specifically what these items really do, how much you need, how to compute your need, the risks involved with over- and under-consumption, and I present specific examples of ads to illustrate the absurdity of the claims made.

Chapter 10, "'Professional' Advice: Who You Can Trust and Who You Can't," is your security blanket. You may feel overwhelmed and insecure about where to go to get a straight answer. This chapter will point you in the right direction by offering helpful resources for additional information.

Chapter 11, "Licensed, Registered, and Certified: Politics, Puffery, or Professional?" uncovers how people use the words "licensed," "registered," and "certified." I'll explain what these terms mean and how a legitimate licensure or certification is acquired.

My discussion of weight-loss programs and products in chapter 12 is vital for all those who believe they need to shed a few or a great many pounds. More than forty million Americans are obese (i.e., they are more than 20 percent over their ideal weight for their sex and height). You'll learn the *only* three *guaranteed* ways to lose weight *permanently*.

Chapter 13 brings the future to the present. With an aging population, this is the new battleground for consumer dollars. Aging "remedies" are exploding. If you're over age thirty-five, you really need to know more about this growing phenomenon. I'll define aging, show you how to slow it down, reverse it, and measure the change—*clinically*, *scientifically*, and *quantitatively*.

Chapter 14 provides valuable "do" and "don't" checklists to insure that you will never be duped again. Your days of being played for a sucker are over!

Do read the glossary. It is a valuable source of information all its own. You might be surprised or even shocked to learn that the phrase "all natural" has no definition. It's a phrase created by manufacturers to attract consumers, but it has no accepted medical or scientific basis. A lot of the terms contained in the glossary were simply invented by marketers to separate you from your money.

I call your attention to features occurring throughout the book.

First you will see boxes that look like this— ☐ —followed by the name I have given to a principle and then some explanatory text. The names of the principles, while somewhat tongue-in-cheek (much like the principles offered in the classic book *The Peter Principle*, by Dr. Laurence Peter), are nonetheless meant to be descriptive labels given to the various methods used to dupe you. These principles are inserted so that you may check them as you read. You check them whenever you come upon a situation or phrase that has led to your being duped. Don't be embarrassed. I checked most of them. I've been duped scores of times. The point is to know that you have been so you can gain the knowledge to prevent future incidents.

The second item is a brief but very important summary at the end of each chapter. The summary is called "VIPs." It stands for "Very Important Points" and contains the information I hope you will remember from each chapter. It is meant to be an easy reference tool and to reinforce your learning.

You should know that I have never endorsed—for compensation or for free—any health or fitness product. I never will. I believe that you are smart enough to make the right choices, if, and only if, you know the truth about the health and fitness industry and how it tries to manipulate you. You don't need me to make recommendations for you. You need this book to learn more about those who want to sell you their products. The truth is the industry's most terrifying nightmare.

You'll see copies of actual ads and Internet addresses. If you find the ad is no longer on the Internet, what might be the reason if the product is supposedly so great?

The objectives of this book are twofold: First, to show you the ways you're being duped—with specific examples and all the subtleties; second, to increase your knowledge so you become self-sufficient and therefore totally competent and able to put misleading and deceptive ads where they belong—in your mental or physical trash bin. I am fully aware you will most likely not have this book with you as you sit at your TV, computer monitor, or with a magazine. Once you learn how and why you're being duped, you most likely will not need it by your side. Knowing a phony ad when you see one reinforces your learning.

Soon, no ad should trick you.

So, dear reader, read, cast aside your ignorance, and grow in knowledge and truth.

I wish you all good health and good fortune.

POWER TO THE SUCKERS!

1 HOW AND WHY YOU GET DUPED
The Head Game

Bluntly, you get duped because you get told what you *want* to hear and shown what you *want* to see. Unfortunately, because the peddlers are so smooth, you oftentimes become an unwitting accomplice and wind up doing the sales job for them and usually you're not even aware of it. You'll see later in this chapter how that happens.

The results are sad—often tragic—and the methods are disgusting.

As much as they want you to believe it, the manufacturers have no personal interest in you. You are seen only as a source of potential revenue.

Make no mistake about it: What the manufacturers do is premeditated, planned, scripted, rehearsed, shot (still or moving pictures), edited, and produced. It is anything but spontaneous.

Being duped is the process whereby you are enticed to purchase something that the manufacturers know—even before you ever see the ad—will not perform as advertised.

What is infuriating to me is that I believe the following should be an absolute requirement of every manufacturer: *The burden of proof should be on the manufacturer or advertiser and not on the consumer.* In reality, it is just the opposite.

By twisting words and phrases, employing the power of implication, creating a definition where there was none, and scores of other tactics, the manufacturers leave it up to you to disprove their claims. They know that this is at best inconvenient and at worst quite difficult. The result? They rake in the bucks while we're left with our frustrations, disappointments, injuries—even death—all the while wasting our money.

Is there anybody out there who is *totally* satisfied with the way they look, the way they feel, and/or their ability to perform a task? Many so-called health and fitness promoters start with the basic premise that the answer to one or more of these questions is no. They then design words, phrases, movements, and even colors to promise you that you can look better, feel better, and perform tasks more effectively and efficiently. They employ the printed word, pictures, and "testimonials" (just to name a few) to reinforce your desire for improvement and to imply or overtly shout that they have the answer to your desires; all at a price in dollars, levels of health and fitness, and sometimes even your life. And it's all staged.

In effect, they prey on your fears, your desires, and your insecurities. Said another way, they believe you are ignorant of the facts and are a sucker.

* * *

It is critical to know how the human body is constructed. This will be evident as we proceed through the chapters. Don't worry. I'm not going to drag you through a course in human anatomy. It's much simpler than that. It takes only seven steps, beginning with the smallest components and progressing through to the complete organism known as the human body. We'll start with atoms and proceed from there. As we build from the smallest element to the end product, we'll proceed through a continuous chain of combination.

When I learned anatomy, we used little "word clues" to remember strings of facts. We did this by making an acronym of the first letter of each word in each level of the chain. For example, the chain below forms the acronym "AMCTOSO." The "S" in the acronym stands for "Systems"; close enough to the whole phrase "Organ Systems." Once the acronym is created, a word is attached to each letter to form some unforgettable mind jogger. Here's what "AMCTOSO" became: All Men Can Talk Of Sports Only. The women loved it because they said that the only thing men talked about was sports. They didn't forget that little ditty. Neither did we. Neither group forgot what the letters then meant in the association with the chain of facts we were trying to memorize.

The chain we will construct looks like this:

ATOMS

⇓

MOLECULES

⇓

CELLS

⇓

TISSUES

⇓

ORGANS

⇓

ORGAN SYSTEMS

⇓

THE ORGANISM

As to the *atoms*, think of the acronym "COHN." That stands for carbon, oxygen, hydrogen, and nitrogen. In combination, they account for approximately 96 percent of the basis of the human body.

Atoms bind together to form *molecules*. For example, combine two atoms of hydrogen and one of oxygen and you get H_2O—water.

Molecules combine to form *cells*. You'll note the word "CELLS" in the above diagram is in bold print. There's a reason for this. It is to draw your attention to that word. *Cells are the basis of life. They are life.* Remember this well: *Everything in this book ultimately relates to cells, whether it's diet, nutrition, digestion, metabolism, exercise, aging, or any other function.*

This is so, because cells contain the living blueprint of your body (your DNA), which determines who you are, what you look like, and, most importantly, how your body responds to and uses vitamins, minerals, supplements, ergogenic aids, and herbs. Inside your cells, you have *genes*. Simply stated, think of them as the computer programs that tell your body what to do, and I mean they tell it *everything*. The science of genetics is derived from that root word "gene." Make no mistake about it; genes play a *large* part in how you respond to anything.

The important point is that everybody's genes are different. Each one of us has anywhere from a small to a very large difference in how we react to any stimulus (lifting weights, eating a pizza, running a mile in eight minutes, etc.). This explains, for example why you and another guy can lift the exact same amount of weights, for the same period of time, and he looks like a linebacker and you still look like a lollipop. No one is sure as to the specific, quantifiable effect that genes have on the physiology (the functioning) of the human body, but there is unanimous agreement that whatever the amount is, it is "a lot." You'll never see or hear the hucksters admit to this basic scientific fact for it would reduce the impact of their message as to what they are trying to sell to you. They want you to believe that everybody can expect the same result. This subtlety will be explained later in this chapter. Go back and read this paragraph. Its importance and your understanding of it cannot be overstated.

Cells combine to form *tissues*, such as skin, the linings of your mouth and stomach, your tendons and ligaments, etc. Tissues combine to form *organs*, such as your eyes, heart, blood vessels, etc. Organs combine to form *organ* systems, such as the heart (cardio) and blood vessels (vascular) to form the cardiovascular system. Combine all the systems and you have just constructed an *organism*, in this case a human being.

Keep this body schematic in mind as you read this book. Again, whatever you do to your body and whatever its action or reaction, it always must ultimately occur at the cellular level. There is no other option.

* * *

Okay, grab your pencil. You're about to have some fun. What follows is what I consider to constitute the fundamentals of fakery. I call them principles and give each a name and number. Check the corresponding box if you've ever been duped that way. Be aware that some are very subtle and you may have been duped, but were not aware of it. They may occur singularly or in combination in any ad. The first principle is the most important. All the others may contain elements of the first one and some that follow may contain elements of others that also follow the first principle.

☐ #1. THE PRINCIPLE OF UNCONSCIOUS IMPLICATION

The Principle of Unconscious Implication means that what you see and/or hear was incomplete but you completed the message the manufacturer wanted you to get. It is here, more than anyplace else, that you are the unwitting accomplice to your own duping.

It is extremely subtle. In effect, you "fill in the blank"—the unstated part of the message—where you may not be aware there even is one.

Here's where you wind up doing the manufacturers' job for them and they don't run the risk of making an obvious phony or unfounded statement.

For example: Assume you're watching your TV and an ad comes on for a piece of exercise equipment for your abdominal muscles. The people in the ad have remarkably well-defined abdominal musculature.

Do they tell you that genetics has a lot to do with their ability to attain that degree of muscular definition? No.

Do they tell you they got that way using *only* that piece of equipment being advertised? Nope.

Do they tell you how long it took to get their level of definition? No way.

Do you know how long it took them to do it? No, you do not.

They may even say something like "In just fifteen minutes a day, you can be on your way to rock-hard abs."What does "on your way" mean? I don't have a clue. Do you?

Do they tell you that you can have very firm abdominal muscles but they are not easily seen? Of course they don't. You may not know it, but you could do five hundred sit-ups a day for a year and still not show the "cuts" (the level of separation between muscles) of the people in the ad. If your abdominal muscles are highly "cut," the front of your stomach looks somewhat like a washboard. Here's why: If you have a lot of fat in your abdominal area, that fat mostly lies between your skin and your abdominal muscles, so the fat "hides" the degree of cut of the abdominal muscles from view, even though you have a pretty "defined" stomach. If you have a very low amount of fat in your abdominal area, you may show the washboard stomach and not even have to do sit-ups or work your abs with any piece of equipment. I hate people with that genetic disposition. Do they tell you how long you must keep up that fifteen-minute-a-day workout to look like them? No.

Do they tell you that the results of whatever time they say to work out with that equipment will result in substantial differences for each individual as to the end result? Not a chance. As an aside, I have never known or heard of any champion bodybuilder who attained their champion-level degree of abdominal definition using those pieces of equipment. Knowing exercise physiology, sport psychology, and athletes as well as I do, I can tell you those bodybuilders would kill to have something that truly worked as well as those abdominal apparatuses with as little effort as is implied.

What you get suckered into doing is making the implication that all you have to do is buy their piece of gear, work out fifteen minutes a day, and in—you fill in the time period yourself—you will have an abdominal area that looks just like the people in the ad.

To continue their charade, the people who are working out during the ad always have great big, continuous smiles on their faces.

The implication is, "Oh, this is the most fun I've had since I was twelve. See how easy and relaxing this is?" They don't say it, but you unconsciously fill in that message. How do you know they don't go out in the parking lot after the taping of the commercial and throw up from localized overexertion? You have no way of knowing what they do after the taping is concluded.

Do you have any idea whether those people have been using anabolic steroids? It may never have entered your mind.

The conclusion that you make is, "If I buy that product, in a short time I'll have the abdominals that look like I've always wanted them to look like." You grab your phone, your credit card, and—congratulations from the manufacturer, sucker—you've just been duped.

☐ #2. THE PRINCIPLE OF SCIENTIFIC TECHNOBABBLE

The Principle of Scientific Technobabble involves the use of words to which you have no clue as to their meaning, but they sound so high-tech and impressive that you assume it's good for you and it must be terribly effective—maybe something you think is on the frontiers of scientific knowledge (for the very reason you *haven't* heard the word or phrase before).

If I said, "This amazing new product is extremely effective in the hyperthermogenic homeostasis of the body's by-product of anabolic exertion," what do you think I'm talking about? I just described an ice cube. All those words just mean somebody got real hot from a heavy dose of exercise and he or she needs cooling off. The purists among you will note that what I said is not exactly correct, but here we go with implication again. You think you know what somebody said but you may be unwilling to admit your ignorance.

The key to deception is to make sure that—except for the most knowledgeable viewer or reader—no one will know the meaning of words and phrases used in an ad.

Another implication you make here is that the words or phrases could not be known to you because, of course, your world is too hectic and, therefore, this really neat manufacturer has spent real money to come up with something that is just too modern and beneficial to pass up. What wasn't even in your vocabulary has just become a necessity.

☐ #3. THE PRINCIPLE OF ANXIOUS ASSOCIATION

The Principle of Anxious Association can work with products or people and usually employs principles 1 and 2, above.

Here's how it works: As to a product, the manufacturer will make the implication that their product is just as good as something else but without harmful side effects. That "something else" may be something that is totally safe, perhaps dangerous, or even blatantly illegal.

Diet-suppression products are one of the most common areas where this occurs. You will hear or see something like this: "Our all-natural, herbal supplements can help you lose weight FAST without the worry or expense of prescription drugs." Most of us who are overweight absolutely do suffer anxiety from that condition. You are searching—anxiously—for a change to that condition and the manufacturer knows it. You are a receptive viewer or listener.

Let's tear this seemingly innocuous ad apart. First, I mentioned before that the phrase "all natural" is meaningless. There is no scientific or medical definition of that phrase. But it's been created by the industry, touted long and loud, and we have accepted it without knowing it is meaningless. The implication here is that it must be "better" because we think it's probably grown without pesticides, manufactured in a completely germ-free environment, and just hangs all over nature waiting to be harvested. None of those statements is true.

Second, herbal supplements are unique in that they do not have to be scientifically proven to be effective at *anything*. They are marketed and sold without a prescription because of politics. A lot of money and political pressure has made them exempt from the stringent standards of proof and purity that are required of all prescription drugs. Herbs are considered supplements and their exemption from being approved by the Food and Drug Administration (which must approve all prescription drugs) has created an immense market for those supplements. In effect, herbal ads can say *anything*. Not so with prescription drugs.

The "worry" stated in the ad is really misleading, for the implication is that, by association, you have to worry about prescription drugs. That is true, but only in the sense that anything—and I mean there are no exceptions—can harm you and even kill you if taken in amounts that exceed the body's ability to safely absorb it.

One of the reasons prescription drugs are so expensive is that they must undergo extremely expensive clinical, scientific trials before they can be approved. The approval process can take years. And, even if you get a drug to market, it has a limited economic life to the "creator"—the pharmaceutical company. This is so, because a drug can legally be patented but, once the time of the patent is up, the formula of that drug can be marketed by anybody, even the pharmaceutical company's competitors. Thus, the higher initial price of a drug is partly that way to allow the pharmaceutical company to recoup its research and development costs of that drug as well as those that don't ever make it to market. You might be interested to know that, according to the FDA, only about one in a hundred drugs that initially begin testing ever makes it to market. So one drug has to cover its own costs and those other ninety-nine that never produced a cent of revenue.

In effect, if you purchased the herbal "remedy" described in the ad, you'd wind up self-prescribing. That can be very dangerous. But the ads never say that, do they?

Of course, when you associate weight loss with the word "FAST," that connection drives people into a spending frenzy. Your own mind conjures up just how fast is "fast," but it really starts the anxiety bubbling just below your level of consciousness and sets up frustration in a big way when you are, ultimately, unable to attain the results in the time period you imposed on yourself.

As to people used in the ads, the manufacturers usually employ somebody famous. As an example, let's take one of my favorite athletes, Michael Jordan. Nike made a very rewarding financial move when they were able to hire Michael to do ads for them. It's not too far-fetched to say that most of us would like to be like Mike. In fact, almost those exact words have been used in ads with Mr. Jordan.

Here's a guy who's good-looking, athletic almost beyond belief, articulate, and probably pays more income taxes in one year than my gross income for my whole life. What Nike wants to get across is that you can be like Mike if you'll just buy these shoes.

That's ludicrous. Do you honestly believe that Michael Jordan couldn't jump before he started wearing Nikes? Do you really believe he can do all the things he does on a basketball court simply because of the brand of shoes he wears? Get serious. I truly believe he could still do a flying, 360°, monster jam while wearing your basic wedgie on one foot and a combat boot on the other.

However, we are led to believe (and we do a bit of leading of ourselves) into thinking we can do some of the things Michael can do and, even if it's not at his level (no pun intended), it surely will be an improvement over what we mere mortals are currently able to accomplish. The subtlest message is that of fantasy. The association to that fantasy is that we may truly know we will never be as good as he is, but we can dream, can't we?

The closest that dream comes to reality is owning something tangible that we can wear that is the same as what our idol really wears.

Thus, our anxiety is to be as much like the world-famous person as we can, even if the limit of reality is only a pair of shoes.

☐ #4. THE PRINCIPLE OF PHANTOM CONNECTION

The Principle of Phantom Connection is the usage of a word or words that imply authority, expertise, acceptance, and/or fame. Here's how this one works. Consider an ad that states something is "clinically proven." When you hear or see that phrase you'll probably nod your head in the affirmative and say, "Clinically proven. Oh, that's good. Yep. Must be okay if it's clinically proven." Do you have any idea what clinic they're talking about? You don't, do you? I admit, I don't. Anybody can create a clinic. For all we know, some guy named Irving Schmedlap could have created the Schmedlap Storm Door and Pharmaceutical Clinic, located in his garage in a lower-class suburb of Ouagadougou.

So, you don't know where this clinic is, or what it does. Do you want to put money on how long ago whatever is advertised was "clinically proven"? Six months? Six years? There's no clue.

Pay attention to this one: Do you know exactly *what* was proven? Nobody tells you. In fact, the "clinical proof" could be that the product was proven *not* to work! Read that again and remember that what was proven is not stated. The manufacturers let you nod your head and grant instant acceptance. Don't blame yourself. I told you these guys were slick.

If it was clinically proven, where in the scientific literature has the proof been presented? Pardon me while I roll on the floor, holding my sides and howling with laughter. There is no citation— and never will be—as to where the proof was published because the manufacturer knows the "proof" would get shredded if it ever appeared in front of the scientific community.

I think you see why the connection is a phantom. It looks real, but it's a mirage, a ghost, a nonreality.

Since we're on a roll, what about the ads that include a phrase like "Four out of five doctors recommend. . . ." Oh, this is a real beaut. I ask you, ladies and gentlemen, what's wrong with that statement? After all, doctors are supposed to know everything. And four out of five is near unanimity. Why, that product must be an all-time winner.

Baloney. First of all, how long ago was this alleged survey taken? It doesn't say, does it? Okay, where was it done? The reader or viewer is left totally in the dark. It could have been taken at a rest home where the doctors were the residents, not the professional staff. Just exactly what kind of doctors are these doctors? Medical doctors? Dentists? Veterinarians? Members of the clergy? Ph.D.s? If Ph.D.s, are their Ph.D.s in sports medicine or exercise physiology, or maybe classical music or economics? Again, we are left to fend for ourselves, but the manufacturer could not care less.

Since I just mentioned economics, were these doctors paid to make the recommendation? You know that will almost never be disclosed. "Four out of five" could mean "four out of five who were polled last Thursday. And the other three hundred who were polled the day before thought the product was junk." What the manufacturer is trying to do is connect medical doctors with acceptance and approval. It's your imagination that provides the glue.

It never fails that somebody famous does an ad. Of course, our drool factor skyrockets off the chart. We just can't believe Studly Goodnight wouldn't tell us anything if it weren't the truth.

For the umpteenth time, we get duped. It's even worse if the celebrity endorser is an athlete and is pushing anything to do with sports, health, or fitness. An interesting extension has occurred in the last twenty or so years. That extension has been the logical limit of knowledge of an athlete. With so much media dependent on their continued exposure, athletes have become implied experts on everything from the Y2K problem to world hunger. These perceptions are noted, analyzed, and fed back into the media in the form of endorsements as truth about something you, the "dupee," strain so mightily to believe that athletes have some special knowledge and expertise that they just can't wait to pass on to you. They're no different than politicians.

You may think I'm stretching credibility as to what was *not* stated. I'm not. The law legally allows—but does not require—the manufacturer to state the truth (sometimes), the whole truth (unless a partial truth works better), and nothing but the truth (but leave it out if it won't sell the product). When the glare of free, critical analysis is placed on the ads, the phantom ceases to exist and the truth is exposed.

☐ #5. THE PRINCIPLE OF THE NODDING LEMMING SYNDROME

The Principle of the Nodding Lemming Syndrome focuses on collectivism and affirmation. Collectivism refers to our natural desire to not only belong, but to be accepted. Affirmation is the repeated nodding of the head in the yes movement.

Lemmings are mouselike rodents. They are also called "loons" from which the word "loony" is derived. They are loony because they will literally destroy themselves by following the lemming in front of them over a cliff.

As it applies here, an ad or announcer will say, "We all want to be healthy, don't we? (Nod your head.) We all want to feel better, don't we? (Nod again.) We all want more energy, don't we? (Keep nodding.)" If you want, you can leap up, thrust your fist in the air, and scream "YES!"

The ad or announcer is subtly forming us into a homogenous group, eliciting our affirmative response and leading us to the cliff, all of which we don't usually notice at a conscious level. Here comes the killer. The ad or announcer tells us it or he or she has the answer to those weighty and emotional questions and that they are there to help you. So we follow the crowd, stride confidently and in ignorance over the cliff of truth, sans parachute.

Incidentally, the ad makers used to use negatives like, "You don't want to be sick, do you? You don't want to be lethargic, do you? You don't want to be fat, do you?" For better or worse, they found that the positive and affirmative worked better than the negative, so the negative is pretty much passé.

☐ #6. THE PRINCIPLE OF INSIPID INDEFINITES AND THE SCREAMING SUPERLATIVES

This principle has two parts. The first, that of Insipid Indefinites, employs the use of words such as "more," "less," "better," "longer," and the like. They are indefinite as to quantity. The ad maker lets you determine the amount. It becomes a case of you attaching a *quantitative* amount to a *qualitative* statement. I show you in chapter 3 how you can measure the amount, but the manufacturer probably doesn't know how to do it, and even if he or she did, they're not going to tell you. If they told you how to measure the amount, they would have to state up front how much that amount is, and they don't want to do that because they don't know what the amount is or it is so small that you wouldn't waste money on their product. So they keep the amount of supposed benefit indefinite and let you generate your own concept of the benefit you might receive.

Here are some examples: "Take this supplement three times a day and you'll have more energy." "Try this product and you'll have less fat (less percentage of body fat than you have at present)." "Buy this and you'll look and feel better."

Consider the word "more" in the previous ad. More energy than what? More energy than a hockey puck? More energy than you had last Tuesday? Do you know how much you had last Tuesday and, if so, how did you measure it? Of course, most of us have no idea. So we blithely spend our money on impossible-to-measure promises.

The manufacturers can be really sneaky. For example, a truly correct scientific study could have determined that their product would actually result in an increase in aerobic endurance of 1.2 percent over a six-month period if taken daily for six months. That amount is so small they just substitute "increase your aerobic endurance" for "a 1.2 percent increase" and hope nobody is the wiser, which we usually aren't.

Insipid Indefinites can also relate to various body parts. That may surprise you, but I saw an ad on my TV. I subscribe to Time-Warner cable and it was on cable channel 42, on 16 July 1999 at approximately 10:30 A.M.

It was an ad for "an all-natural herbal alternative to Viagra.™" I believe the product was spelled X-e-n-e-r-e-l. During this ad, a gentleman came on who was identified by words on the screen that were "Stephen Baker, M.D., Internal Medicine." The good doctor stated that the way this product worked was to "vasodilate [it means to open up blood vessels to increase blood flow] specific parts of your body." Hmmmm, he never said what those body parts were. Is it a secret? Gee, Dr. Baker, when I studied anatomy, we used to identify body parts. I could look at a picture and say, "Yep, that's a foot." I have no idea what herbs are contained in this product or what body parts are affected.

If you ever encounter a screaming superlative, turn the page, switch the channel, tune to another station, stuff earplugs in your ears. Do not—I repeat—do *not* give any credence whatsoever to any ads that contain the following words:

- Amazing
- Incredible
- Remarkable

- Revolutionary
- Extraordinary
- Exclusive
- Fabulous
- Astonishing
- Effortless
- Stunning
- Secret formula
- Guaranteed
- Fantastic
- Unbelievable
- Miraculous

Of course, I could list scores more. We've all heard or read them.

I want you to do something. I want you to take your pencil and write in what you think is the definition of "incredible." No fair looking in a dictionary. You have fifteen seconds. Go ahead and write your definition in the following space:

_____

_____

Time's up. The definition of incredible is "so extraordinary as to seem impossible."

That definition was taken from my *Random House Dictionary of the English Language*, unabridged edition. Think about that definition for a moment. Have we not used words so many times that we have diluted not only their meaning but also their impact? I contend we have. So what the manufacturers do is increase the size of those words in print relative to the size of the surrounding print, increase the volume of the speaker reading the ad lines, or combine many of the screaming superlatives so as to try for the "multiplier effect"— putting several in the same ad thereby overwhelming you and crushing your resistance. And you get duped yet again.

I have known a guy for over thirty years who is a "biggie in the ad biz" as he likes to say. We were classmates at Notre Dame over thirty years ago. He requested anonymity for what follows: he told me if his name were used in connection with what follows he'd get a rap as a "rat" and it could cost him his company. I take his request seriously and will honor it.

I asked his assistance in dissecting a TV ad for a typical product in the health and fitness industry. What he told me was how the ad maker uses various devices and methods to get a point across to separate you from your money. Let's take a fascinating look inside the ad industry and see how ad makers do this. Some of the comments and conversation are mine, as I can't resist interjecting some caustic humor into the whole process.

He says that the first thing manufacturers will do is to decide what product they want to market. It can be a new product or placing increased emphasis on an existing product if there appears to be increased public interest or awareness due to an externality.

An example of an externality would be the supplement androstenedione (an-droh-STEEN-die-own). This really became notorious because of the baseball player Mark McGwire. In 1998, when he was clobbering monstrous home runs at a record pace, it was learned he took this supplement. The supplement industry went nuts. If a supplement manufacturer wasn't manufacturing it, that was changed in a hurry. If a manufacturer was already manufacturing it, that manufacturer put a whole new advertising emphasis on it.

Once the product has been selected, the next step is to create the ad campaign. (To "Big Mac's" credit, I know of no instance where he endorsed "andro." In fact, as of August 1999, he announced on ESPN that he had quit taking "andro" more than four months earlier and had no intention of taking it again. He said he had heard that too many young kids were taking it, thinking the pills alone would make them hit homers. He said the claims made about "andro" just were not true.) The ad campaign then progresses to the market(s) to which the ad will be directed. Market(s) means you and me—the consumers.

It gets quite precise, and is done by a process known as stratification. For example, say the manufacturer wants to sell a product that is suitable only for women. Stratification means to subdivide into smaller units. So the manufacturer may decide to market the product to women, who are married, between the ages of forty and sixty, with incomes above $30,000 per year.

Then the form of media is selected. Media refers to TV, radio, magazines, newspapers, etc. It is here that the cost of the time and space needed to present the ad is computed and compared against the budget.

Concurrently, the market location is selected. The location is geographic, such as only English-speaking countries, like the United States, Australia, and the United Kingdom. It could also be restricted to Sun Belt states within the United States. The lawyers check and see if there are any administrative (legal) reasons preventing the sale in given locations.

Then the ad is scripted and edited. Here's where all the words and phrases to be used are written and rewritten until the expected desired message is created. It is also where elements so specific as colors to be used in the ad; the props to be included; and location for printing, recording, or filming are determined.

Then the actors and actresses are hired. In some cases, "real people" are used, to imply they are no different from us. Sometimes, famous people are hired to present their testimonial, their value being one of instant recognition.

Regardless of who is employed for the task, a producer and/or production coordinator has to bring all the elements together, not the least being the communications system to make it oh-so-convenient for you to buy the product (800 numbers, credit cards accepted, operators standing by).

The lines and movements are memorized, rehearsed, shot (with an average of between forty to sixty "takes" for a single, one-minute TV ad not unusual), edited, produced, and finally placed on the air.

If someone will hand me my scalpel, we'll create a mental image of a typical TV ad and I'll dissect it and hold up the elements for you to see. Keep this in mind when you next see an ad on TV.

First, notice the coloring and background. The colors are usually pastels because they are nonoffensive to most people. Seldom are the dark colors of black, purple, blue, red, and green used. They supposedly denote sorrow, "heaviness," a barrier. The background may be a bookcase, nice wallpaper or paint on the walls, a few lamps and pictures, but nothing that appears cluttered. There should be no background shadows and the lighting should especially complement the individuals used in the ad.

Those individuals must appear to be intelligent, healthy, energetic, attractive, have great bodies, etc. You know what I'm talking about.

Both the guys and girls must have professional makeup artists do their hair and faces and, sometimes, their bodies. My friend says, "We 'do a Hugh' on 'em," meaning substantial touching up à la Hugh Hefner for the photos in *Playboy*. What you see is somebody who has perfectly coiffured hair, tan from a tube, exactly the right amount of "stage sweat" (a watery substance sprayed on the body to look like perspiration), capped teeth, no skin blemishes or pockmarks. The clothes must be just on the borderline of being "suggestive" (sexually appealing and revealing). Sometimes they go way over that line.

The positioning of the individuals is critical. This is usually the case of the "nonexistent interviewer." What happens here is that, say, a female is seated and looking just to the left or right of the camera lens, giving the appearance that she is answering a question that has just been posed to her about this all-natural, exciting, revolutionary, amazing, unbelievable, remarkable new product (and clinically proven, don'tcha know). What she's really doing is looking at a prompter with her lines on them. In a few cases it may be a mirror so she can see herself, to make sure her head is erect, she's not blinking too much, she continues to talk through smiling teeth, etc.

She has this attitude that "I am just so bouncy and perky" (yeah, and if her smile got any wider, her face would fall off). But she has this oh-so-sincere look of credibility and appreciation and says something ridiculous like, "Well, only three months ago I weighed over three hundred pounds and had no money and no energy. But then I heard about this really, like, y'know, incredible discovery by Dr. Forness that promised me a handsome hunk of man, abundant riches, and the secret of life so I bought a sixty-day supply and in no time at all the results were unbelievable. They were incredible. In no time at all I had more energy, I lost weight, and I became more physically fit. It was all so fast and easy! And I did it all in the privacy of my own home! You should really get this product. It will work wonders for you in no time at all!"

A slight variation is where there actually is an interviewer. Their lines are usually few. But if you notice closely, they usually have a notebook propped on their knee and, whenever the camera is on them, they have their chin resting on the "Y" formed by the tips of their thumb and forefinger and they are always nodding sagely in the affirmative direction. The implication is that they understand and are agreeing with what she is saying.

I asked my industry source if they coached the interviewer about nodding. "You bet we do. We coach them on how far to nod the head. Never want them nodding so far that eyes cannot be seen. We coach them on how fast to nod their heads. We coach them to always have a 'receptive' look on their face. It would never do to have an 'interviewer' nodding in the affirmative while grimacing. You never want more than one message at a time from body language when you're doing an ad like that."

Another subtle implication is that the woman has just heard the doorbell ring, answers the door, and twenty-six people and cameras crash in, but she is not at all awed or curious as to how they found her. In fact, she looks totally nonplussed and the scene is meant to exhibit normalcy. The implication here is that the whole staged scene is actually complete and utter spontaneity.

The guy may then come on and, nearly faint from three hours of weightlifting to get just the right pump in his muscles, he at once tries to look relaxed while flexing so hard his veins are ready to pop. He is striving mightily for that relaxed yet taut look as if to imply his muscles are pumped like that even while sleeping.

"That's right, Baby, this product was clinically proven to be safe and effective. It's recommended by four out of five doctors. Why, its herbal ingredients don't have any side effects. It's guaranteed effective. And, if you call right now, you can get a lifetime supply for only $18,995. If you are among the next 100 callers we'll even throw in another lifetime supply absolutely free. That's a $2,000,000 value! (Who's counting?) Folks, you can't afford to pass up this amazing offer. Just get your credit card and call *right now*. Operators are standing by. We want to hear from you right now! The number to call is 1-800-U-SUCKER. That's 1-800-U-SUCKER!"

Want to have some more fun? Go back and cross out with your pencil everything that the guy and the gal said that you feel is misleading and/or fraudulent. Go ahead. I'll just sit here and wait for you and hum a few bars of "Lies, Lies, and More Lies."

Okay. Welcome back. The only parts that should not have been crossed out were the sentences having to do with the operators standing by and the (fictitious) phone number. Everything else is phony. If you did cross out everything but what I just mentioned, you're on your way to becoming a pro at "ad busting."

*   *   *

Even when the ad is over, the machines of capitalism are still running full force. Once you make that purchase, your name, address, phone number, and credit card are now known, as well as the product you just purchased. What the manufacturer does is sell that information to mailing list companies who then sell your information to anybody who wants to buy that information. Now you may know why, in the months after you buy a product, you start getting unsolicited telephone calls, mailers, and the like to buy a similar or associated product.

You may also notice something on the screen in small print. Something to the effect of "Please allow 6–8 weeks for delivery." What's that all about? What it is about is that the manufacturers generally have no solid idea how much increase in demand—if any—will result as a consequence of the ad. Therefore, what they do is a procedure called "batch processing." Batch processing is taking and saving all the orders during a specific period—say thirty days—and then those orders are filled all at once. Temporary workers are hired to fill the increase in orders and then let go.

The means by which products are sold has changed rather dramatically in the last twenty years. For instance, supplements were first sold primarily in what we used to call drugstores. Then they began being offered in magazines and supermarkets. Then they expanded to health-food stores. Then they began being sold via multilevel marketing firms. And now you have an uncountable amount of sales being made via the Internet.

Multilevel marketing (MLM) is like love: easy to know but hard to define. The difficulty arises when MLM is compared to what is known as "pyramiding." Pyramiding was initially a process used in the securities industry by investors. What they would do is buy a stock on margin; that is, only paying part of the selling price and having

the broker borrow the rest. Then, hopefully, as the price of the purchased stock rose, it would have more value that the investor could
borrow against, use the borrowed funds to buy more stock on
margin, and keep repeating the cycle. All is great until the price of
the stock drops, then the broker issues margin calls—demands to
come up with cash by the investor. If the investor didn't have the
cash, the whole pyramid would collapse—which is just what happened in the stock market in 1929.

This concept got bastardized into meaning any individual or company that would buy something like real estate (sometimes inside a
limited partnership, sometimes not) and use the same borrowed
money idea, except the money was borrowed by the syndicators
from the investors in the scheme. Eventually, the hucksters who set
up the pyramid would disappear, leaving the investors with a ton of
debt and the property would be lost.

The visual concept of a pyramid is valid as it relates to MLM.
You've got very few people at the top and a huge amount at the lower
levels of the pyramid. The idea is that everybody at the levels above
gets a percentage of everything that is sold by the people in all the
levels below. In the area of health and fitness products, the concept
is manipulated so that the majority of the sales are made to the salespeople themselves, and not to customers! The salespeople are
required to purchase "sales kits" which include a certain amount of
the product to be sold to the consumer. MLM is valid in concept. Any
organization, whether it be IBM, Gateway Computer, General
Motors, Shaklee, or anybody else is entirely legal in setting up an
organization where the people higher up get a percentage of what
the people at the levels below sell to the customer. The "higher-ups"
get a percent of all sales whether or not the sale is made to a "rep"
below them, or to a customer who is not a rep. By requiring reps to
buy a certain amount, this *guarantees* a commission to every higher-
up, even if the rep never sells a single item to a customer. It also puts
pressure on the reps to hire reps under them (the "down line") so the
hiring reps (the "up line") make money.

All too often, the sales people at the lower levels are basically
ignorant as to the real benefits and risks of what they are selling. Many
MLM companies have also been nailed by the law because they have

required their sales people—who are really not employees at all but independent representatives (also known as independent contractors)—to pay just to become a "rep" and thereafter to pay an amount periodically (usually annually) to continue to be a rep and to receive a percentage of the sales of those they recruit—called the "down line."

This all virtually shouts "Let the buyer beware." When I was studying law, I remember reading that, in addition to caveat emptor, there was a companion phrase "caveat vendor" which means "let the seller beware." About six hundred years ago, both phrases were applicable because people bargained for goods and services with people they knew personally. Caveat emptor and caveat vendor implied the current phraseology of "a level playing field." Effectively, because of the barter economies that existed at that time, neither the buyer nor the seller could attain an unfair advantage over the other (at least for very long).

About one hundred years later, the consumer had acquired so much power that it was the *vendor* who had to beware, not the consumer. At the turn of the twentieth century and for approximately forty years thereafter, caveat emptor became more and more the guiding principle. In fact, the issue of whether the vendor or the consumer has the ultimate responsibility for the truth of an ad about a product or service went as high as the U.S. Supreme Court.

Thus, the market situation today places more burden of proof as to efficacy and legitimacy of all goods and services on the *consumer* than at any time in this country's history.

Last, you may or may not have heard of a word called "puffery." Puffery is allowed by law. It is the use of words or phrases by the seller that should not be taken as material to the sale. An example would be the friendly used-car salesman who says, "I got the cleanest cars in the county." He may not know that factually, or it may be an outright lie, but the law says that that type of phrase is not what entices the buyer to buy, so it is allowed in the sales pitch. The line between puffery and deception may not be static and it may not be clear.

How'd you like to see a real ad that contains most of the principles I've previously stated? (You will see a lot, lot more, especially in chapters 4 through 9. These are not my creations. They come directly to you from the manufacturers and sellers.)

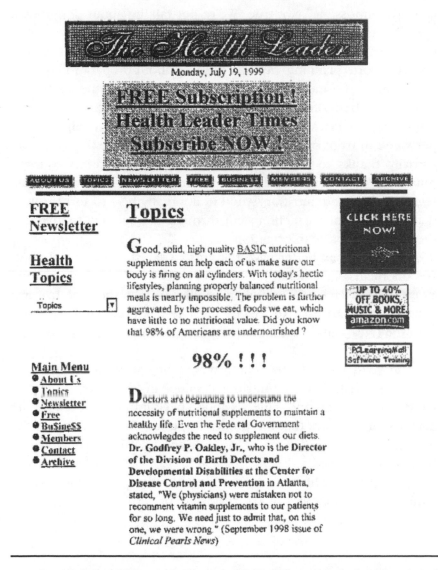

On 19 July 1999 at 12:51 P.M. (EDT) I downloaded and printed an ad from the *Health Leader* at its Internet address http://www. healthleader.com/topics.htm (page 1 of 3). Take a look at that ad. Start with the paragraph under the word "**TOPICS**" and note how it hits you with "today's hectic lifestyles." I call your attention to that phrase in the paragraph immediately preceding principle 3. The ad goes on to state that "planning properly balanced nutritional meals

is nearly impossible." Not true. We're not talking about designing a space shuttle. The ad implies that it's just so difficult to do anything in our "hectic lifestyles"—even planning what we eat. And notice it uses the word "planning" but says nothing about preparation or consumption of the meal. Why not? It's because what the ad sells is assumed to be lacking in your meal planning. Did you know that the average American now spends an average of twenty-eight hours per week in front of a TV set? What a hectic lifestyle that must be. Partially thanks to the Internet and distance education courses, Americans have an unparalleled amount of information available regarding diet and nutrition. And I'm doing my best to sort through that information avalanche to cut through the baloney to give you the nonhyped basic information.

Somebody had better have the guts to say something. I'll do it: We Americans, in general, are lazy apologists and create straw men to excuse our lack of exercise and ability to take the time to learn what we need to eat. No, hectic lifestyle has precious little to do with the (false) implication that we just don't have time to care for a basic necessity.

The vendors really get rolling when they state that "processed foods . . . have little or no nutritional value." In fact, most processed foods have vitamins and minerals added back into them because the manufacturer knows that the processing does, in fact, result in the diminishing or loss of some of the nutrients that existed before the processing occurs.

Then these ads hit you with the big lie in large, bold font, no less: "Did you know that 98% of Americans are undernourished?

98%!!!"

I have no idea where they came up with that figure. I don't know about you, but the implication you are supposed to get is that we Americans are undernourished across the board—in every vitamin and mineral, plus fiber, amino acids, etc., etc., and etc. Is that what came to mind when you read it? It's nothing but a scare tactic.

Incidentally, "undernourished" is like "all natural" in that it does not have a scientific or medical definition. "Undernutrition" does;

"undernourished" does not. So, if you can't define it, you can't identify it or determine how many people are above or below it. (Clue:
The manufacturer wants you to put your own definition into that
implication of the word.)

Then the ad goes on to state that "Doctors are beginning to understand the necessity of nutritional supplements to maintain a healthy
life." Ladies and gentlemen, you may be interested to know that the
first vitamin was discovered over eighty years ago. Do you mean to
tell me we're just beginning to study this whole situation? Why, I
remember talking with Dr. Robert Kerlan, M.D., a sports medicine
pioneer in Los Angeles, almost thirty years ago, about nutrition. Dr.
Kerlan really knew nutrition inside out. And over fifty years ago
scores of medical studies were done on Americans who were taken
as POWs by the Japanese in World War II, and were studied inten-
sively as to their health and nutrition problems while being held cap-
tive. Other studies were done on soldiers—primarily U.S. Marines—
who fought in that same war in the South Pacific campaigns and who
were subject to scores of diseases and malnutrition while fighting
and being undersupplied by our own logistics in the jungles of those
Pacific islands. We have known about the value of vitamins and minerals in our daily diet for decades.

As the ad continues, it throws a sneak punch when it says, "Even
the Federal Government acknowledges the need to supplement our
diets." Technically that's true. In fact, most health and medical practitioners know it to be true. However, it's not—repeat *not*—on the
implied, all-pervasive basis the ad wants you to believe. You see, we
know that in extremely limited situations some Americans need to
supplement their diets. Here's an example: A woman *might* need to
supplement her iron intake during her pregnancy. Nothing amazing
about that fact. It's widely known. The ad maker wants you to
believe we *all* need to supplement our diets. That is not true.

The implication is that the federal government has been hiding this
bit of knowledge (probably next to the files entitled "Who Really Killed
JFK" and "Where We Hid the UFOs"). The implication seems to be that
the federal government has somehow, mysteriously, been caught in a
cover-up and just as mysteriously been forced to reveal its secrets.

What a load of hogwash.

VIPS

Everything you do to your body affects it at the cellular level.

Implication, with you the consumer completing the thought, is the most powerful tool used by the manufacturers.

The ads are incredibly subtle, with copious phrasing that is misleading, indefinite, and unconnected.

The burden of proof as to the legitimacy of any ad is on you the consumer, not on the producer.

In the next chapter I'll show you how anything that is claimed to be "scientifically proven" can, in fact, be proven as true and how it can be proven as false.

2 THE SCIENTIFIC METHOD
How to Prove What *Is* the Truth

I think thcrc's a strange disease that afflicts people in the health and fitness industry. I don't know if it has a name. You may have seen someone with the symptoms.

If I had to guess, I think they could contract it in the following manner: You're browsing in a health-food store. A person walks in and strides up to "Harold," the sales clerk, and says, "I want to buy some protein. It has to be in powdered form; not granulated. It must be at least 90 percent anhydrous."

Harold thinks, *Uhhhh, man, I don't need this. What is this andy hydro, er . . . hydrant . . . uh, whatever.* Trying to regain his composure, Harold leads the customer over to an area he hopes contains protein while simultaneously attempting to do a speed-reading on the labels and packaging to see if what has been requested is in stock.

With an incredible stroke of luck, he locates a powdered protein product that is 90 percent anhydrous. "Here ya go, pal. Just what you wanted."

The customer says, "Very good. Please show me the scientific citations that support the claims made on the label for this product."

Suddenly, Harold's eyes start to flash and roll back in his head, his breathing becomes labored, he staggers around the store in spastic motions, and his words are unintelligible. Whatever this affliction is, I hope it's not endemic or contagious.

The bottom line is that there are no scientific citations because the supporting scientific studies relative to the claims of the product have never been done. Since they haven't been done, they've never been published in any legitimate scientific journals. Isn't it curious how the manufacturers and sellers of health and fitness products want you to take everything *they* say on faith and as unquestionably true, but can't produce the truth to back up their claims?

There is one way—and one way only—to prove whether the claims that are made are true or not. It is called the scientific method. *When something has been proved using the scientific method, it is said to have been "scientifically proven" or "proven scientifically."* No other option is possible or allowed. This scientific proof is really "how we know what we know." It is something that is at once reliable, consistent, universal, and unassailable. It is the *truth*.

*   *   *

Grab your pencil and I'll show you the results of some studies that have been proved by the scientific method, then I'll explain how it works. You'll note below that there are eleven statements. Each statement has a line and a number to the left of it. There are no trick statements. I present them as plainly as possible. What I want you to do is read a statement. After you've read it, put a "1,""2," or "3" just above the line next to that statement's number.

Put a "1" if you believe the statement has been scientifically proven *not* to be true for the general population. In other words, the statement can be said to be *universally false*.

Put a "2" if you believe the statement has been scientifically proven to be true, but only in *limited* studies or *limited* applications.

Put a "3" if you believe the statement has been scientifically proven to be true for the general population. In other words, the statement can be said to be *universally true*.

____ 1. Approximately 10 percent of your daily caloric intake is used up merely digesting the food and drink you ingested.

___ 2. Taking vitamin supplements prolongs your life.

___ 3. Vitamins can replace food.

___ 4. The human brain runs out of storage space after age forty-five.

___ 5. If you lift weights for many years and suddenly stop, the extra muscle you gained will eventually turn to fat.

___ 6. Vitamin C can prevent certain kinds of cancer.

___ 7. Grapefruit has been proven not to increase or decrease your metabolism.

___ 8. A person will not gain weight if he or she eats only nonfat foods.

___ 9. Low vitamin E levels have been linked to memory loss.

___ 10. A woman who takes estrogen supplements may wind up with an increased bust size.

___ 11. No vitamins have ever been proven to either produce or increase energy in the human body.

I must iterate that there is no trickery intended or used in any of the statements. Every one of them has been scientifically proven to be the actual answer as given below.

1. The answer is "3." Scientific studies have consistently shown that, while there are small variations in the amount, the mean (arithmetic average) is, in fact, 10 percent.

2. The answer is "1." There has never been a single scientific study that proved any single vitamin, or combination of vitamins, can prolong your life.

3. The answer is "1." In fact, vitamins cannot be assimilated by the body without ingesting food. That is why you are correctly advised to take vitamins with a meal.

4. The answer is "2." A recent study published in the journal *Developmental Psychology* (July 1999) on 778 subjects showed that the brain seems to have the ability to continue to store information without incurring a problem of storage space up to age forty-five, after which it declines. Be careful: A "2" means that, while the statement is correct, it has only been shown to be as stated in a *limited* study or application. It is not yet widely proven to apply to the general population.

5. The answer is "1." This "old wives' tale" just won't go away. Fat is not muscle. Muscle is not fat. One will never, ever, turn into the other, regardless of what you do or don't do. Recall what we did in the first chapter when we built the human body. At the cellular level you have fat cells and you have muscle cells (among others). They keep their identity throughout their whole existence—your entire life.

6. The answer is "1." There is some evidence that vitamins C and E may combat (prevent) the spread or growth of a tumor, but this refers to a situation *after* the cancer has reached a given level of development. They have never been proven as a cancer preventive. The greatest proponent of vitamin C as a preventive of cancer, the common cold, and certain mental illnesses and other illnesses was Dr. Linus Pauling. Unfortunately, though he took massive doses of vitamin C, his ultimate legacy is tarnished. He died of cancer in 1994. His wife also died of cancer.

7. The answer is "3." Grapefruit has been touted by hucksters as a great weight-loss aid because, they claim, it "naturally increases your metabolism, which speeds weight loss." Not only has grapefruit never been proven to increase your metabolism, it has never been proven to decrease it.

8. The answer is "1." Another example of an incorrect belief that won't die. Other than water, virtually everything we eat or drink has some fat content to it. For example, you may see some pasta advertised as "nonfat." However, pasta is a form of carbohydrate. Carbohydrates will be converted to fat if the body does not utilize them quickly enough. In fact, your body needs a certain amount of fat to lubricate your joints, aid in hormone production, act as an insulator against cold, etc.

9. The answer is "2." The studies which have shown this have been done only on people age sixty and older. Also, the subjects who exhibited the greatest memory loss were those who skipped entire meals and/or who had inadequate nutrition as recommended by professionals for their age, gender, and activity level.

10. The answer is "2." Ladies, don't go out and buy up all the estrogen. Limited studies have shown that women who had

estrogen levels *below* that recommended for their age, whether they were pre- or postmenopausal and were pregnant or not at the time of the study, did show an increase in bust size when they took supplemental estrogen. When the estrogen levels were then increased to the recommended levels, it was found that the bust size increase was very small. Sorry.

11. The answer is "3." This ranks right up there with the muscle/fat and vitamin/longevity misconceptions as given above. While vitamins are unquestionably necessary for life, in and of themselves they neither produce nor increase energy in the human body.

The manufacturers are generally aware of whether their product would be a number 1, 2, or 3. Knowing this, they continue to deceive you. This deception can be stated as another principle.

☐ #7. THE PRINCIPLE OF EXPERIMENT EXTENSION

The Principle of Experiment Extension works like this: The manufacturer knows that his product is a number 2. He doesn't state it that way. He takes the results of a scientific experiment in a limited study or one that that has shown limited application and tries to get you to believe that it is really a number 3—that it has universal application to the general population.

To illustrate, take the question and answer to number 4, above. The manufacturer will state something like, "The human brain loses its ability to store additional information after you reach age forty-five." Then the manufacturer will tout its product, that has been shown to have very limited application, and say, "Buy our (name of product). It has been clinically proven to increase your memory." Of course, when you tie the two statements together, you're led to believe that you can increase your brain's ability to continue to add information, especially if you're over age forty-five, if only you'll buy the product. Nowhere in the ad does it say that those two statements have very limited application, nor does it state how much the increase is. Don't get suckered by this tactic.

But the manufacturers can get even more sophisticated in their methods. As an addendum to the above, they may even list several articles from respected scientific journals that appear to support their claims. This is really tough to resist. But, if you had access to these articles, and were skilled enough to read and understand what the experiments and studies found in fact, you would know that these almost always fall into the number 2 category.

Then advertisers may do something that is so subtle you probably would never be aware of it. The manufacturer has taken these studies, which relate to some, but usually not all of the ingredients in their product, and duped the consumer by implication. The implication is either: (a) the studies they cite refer to the product as a whole, or (b) the studies collectively result in universal application. Then they will create the "grabbers"—the words and phrases that really get your attention—to tout the product and get you to buy it.

Some manufacturers are so good, they can combine most of the principles that I have already stated. The ads can be extremely powerful. It is hard to resist them, even if you may be a little skeptical. Too often you overcome your own skepticism and buy the product with an attitude of, "Well, I really don't believe what they say, but I guess it can't hurt to at least give it a try." I can only respond to that attitude by wondering that if you really don't believe what they say, why are you buying the product? What is in the following illustration is a perfect example of this. (You should know that, because of my professional standing I receive a tremendous number of ads and magazines through the regular mail. I deliberately request some; many of them come unsolicited. The reason I continue to read them is to keep up on what the hucksters are doing. By requesting them and/or merely continuing to receive them, I in no way endorse the product[s] advertised.)

The folks at Gero Vita International sent me a sixteen-page ad, which I received on 22 July 1999. The front cover is the illustration (below) and the scientific study citations are listed on the following illustration page, which is page 11 of their ad. Look at the first illustration page. The ad promises to allow you to "breathe easier . . ." (though it doesn't tell you easier than what). It almost defies belief when it continues (as one example) ". . . and end . . . heart problems." It doesn't say what those specific heart problems are, does it?

The second illustration page lists twelve citations. It's a lot of small print and big words. Read the titles of those citations. Do you really know what they mean? Even if you can understand the big words, do you know the results of each study?

I took the entire ad and found it violated every one of the seven principles I've stated so far.

The media is the greatest friend of the manufacturers. It tries to grab your attention with pictures, words, or sound bites. These are very short, dynamic, emotional pieces of a story that you just must read, listen to, or watch. I fully expect some announcer to come on TV and scream, *"End of the world tomorrow! Film at eleven. . . .* And now for the five-day weather forecast . . ."

Try something. Go back and look at question 6. What kind of sound bite could you create for that? I think I'd create, "Study shows vitamin C prevents cancer." When you're done creating the sound bite, read again the answer to number 6 and you'll learn, if you haven't already, how someone can twist or spin the truth and not tell the whole story.

I think you're ready to learn the specifics of the scientific method. To keep it simple for you, I'll list the simplest version of the scientific method:

1. State the problem (observation and description of a phenomenon from the physical universe);

2. Form a hypothesis (statement as to why this phenomenon occurs, and what might be done to change it. This is speculation at this point);

3. Use the hypothesis to make a prediction as to what the expected outcome of the experiment is likely to be;

4. Test the hypothesis and determine, quantitatively and by observation, whether the hypothesis is true or not.

I'll now expand on each step and give you more details and examples to help you further understand the process.

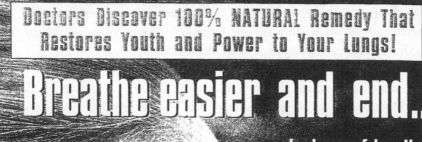

Doctors Discover 100% NATURAL Remedy That Restores Youth and Power to Your Lungs!

Breathe easier and end..

...shortness of breath
...smoking damage
...chest congestion
...heart problems
...sinus problems
...colds & flu
...emphysema
...bronchitis
...allergies
...fatigue
...asthma

Safe
No Drugs
No Side Effects

1. You look at the physical universe. ("Universe" does not necessarily imply the entire solar system. It can mean something of this world—and usually does.) For example, you observe sedentary adults in the Atlanta area and it appears to you that many of them have high percentages of body fat. You have also observed that weightlifters who take dehydroepiandrosterone (DHEA) have very low percentages of body fat. You don't know what amount of the low body-fat percentage in weightlifters is due to weightlifting and what amount is due to DHEA, which is reputed to lower percent body fat and increase muscle mass.

2. Your hypothesis might be that you think DHEA might lower percent body fat in otherwise sedentary adults, even if they do not lift weights. You believe this to be true because you know DHEA is an androgenic substance—one that causes muscularization. Because you can find no scientific studies on the effect of DHEA on sedentary adults, you decide to conduct an experiment to determine what, if any effect, DHEA has on the level of percent body fat in sedentary adults.

3. You predict that a sedentary adult (which you define as being between the ages of forty and sixty years, and who exercises less than two hours per week) will experience a 10 percent reduction of percent body fat if that person takes 50 mg of DHEA daily for ninety consecutive days.

4. In testing your hypothesis, you must set up the experiment. To do this, you need to do several things. First, you have to select the subjects that will be part of the experiment. This is done by the process known as "random sampling."

   Because you cannot study every sedentary adult in the United States (it would take too long and cost too much money), you select a small percentage of them to study. All sedentary adults in the United States are called the "population" and the ones selected for your study are called the "sample." In making the random sample (selection), you want to make sure that the sample is representative of the population.

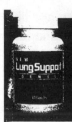

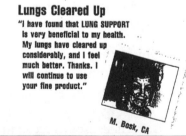
In other words, the sample should be a cross-section of the population—the individuals selected should have the same *essential* characteristics as the population. The essential characteristics in this example might be that those selected cannot be active, weightlifters, taking DHEA; must be

between forty and sixty years of age; and have no health or medical conditions that preclude them from taking DHEA.

Random sampling means that each member of a population has an equal chance of being selected. This is the only kind of sample that can ensure the selection process is free of bias. Bias means including individuals in the sample who are known to possess characteristics that will favorably or unfavorably influence the results of the experiment—and these characteristics are known *before* the experiment is performed. Consider bias as "stacking the deck" of the experiment.

Assume you want to study two hundred sedentary adults in the Atlanta area. You randomly select them from the population in the Atlanta area, and you actually can do this by advertising for volunteers, and then screening them to see that each meets the criteria—the essential characteristics, as mentioned above—to be included.

Is there anything magical about the number being two hundred? No, but historically the results of experiments that had fewer than thirty subjects have not been given much credence. The reason is that fewer than thirty subjects has been mathematically shown to be too few to differentiate significant differences in the results. Any good text on statistical methodology or statistical inference will verify this.

Next, you divide the two hundred subjects into two groups of one hundred people each. One group is known as group A, the other as group B. You perform a percent body-fat test on each and every subject immediately before the experiment is to begin. This is most cost-effectively done by using what is known as a "skinfold caliper." A skinfold caliper is a noninvasive instrument that measures in millimeters the amount of skin and subcutaneous (below the skin) fat on a person. The most common protocol is what is known as the "sum of 9-skinfold measurements," as has been used by the American College of Sports Medicine and its members for more than thirty years.

The caliper is positioned on nine areas of the body—the tricep, thigh, abdominal, chest/pectoral, medial calf, midaxillary, subscapular, suprailium, and biceps area. (For the specific locations on the body, see: *Resource Manual for Guidelines for Exercise Testing and Prescription*, 2d edition, by the American College of Sports Medicine [Baltimore: Williams and Wilkins, 1993], pp. 11–14.) The skinfold caliper, especially a good one such as the Lange Skinfold Caliper, will come with a table so you can convert the measurements into percent body fat and percent lean mass.

The testing that is done immediately before the experiment is done is called the "pretest," and is done to establish the beginning values of percent body fat for each subject. *It is critically important that the subjects be told that they must make no changes in diet or lifestyle during the experiment. This is done so as to make certain that any change in percent body fat is solely due to the DHEA, and nothing else.*

Group A will be given the DHEA and group B will be given the placebo. A placebo is a completely inert pill/capsule. It has no active ingredients. It does nothing—good or bad—for the subject. In this experiment, it looks just like the DHEA pill. However, to further guarantee that the experiment is free from bias, no one in group A or group B knows which capsule he or she is getting. In fact, the person who gives the capsule to each subject does not know the difference. Both the real capsule and the placebo look and taste alike.

This dispensing of the capsules is known as a "double-blind." It means neither the subjects nor the person dispensing the capsules knows which is real and which is the placebo. How does anybody know which is which? The answer is that the person who distributes the capsules to the one who administers them to the subjects *does* know. For example, person Y takes the DHEA capsules and gives them to person Z, who administers them to group A, while both persons, Y and Z, observe that all the subjects in group A do, in fact, swallow the capsules. The same procedure is performed with group B, except those subjects get the placebo. The experiment continues for ninety consecutive days, at which time no more capsules are administered and each subject has his or her percent body fat tested. This is called the "posttest." At the end of the posttest, both group A and group B have taken nothing for thirty days. This is known as the "washout period," which is the time it takes for all traces and effects of the DHEA to reach zero. The second phase of testing occurs, exactly the same as the first phase, except this time group B takes the DHEA and group A takes the placebo.

When this second phase is completed, you compare the results of each stage on each group. What you are hoping to observe is that, in the first stage, each person in group A has experienced a 10 percent reduction of body fat and each person in group B has had no reduction in percent body fat. You further hope that these results are reversed in the second phase. If you get these results, you can say that the reason percent body fat was decreased by 10 percent in each individual was due to the daily intake of 50 mg of DHEA. In reality you should not expect each person to have a reduction of exactly 10 percent, but if the *average* of all scores is 10 percent, you have made a significant discovery.

The entire process I have just presented to you is called a "random-selection, two-phase, pretest/posttest, placebo-controlled, double-blind, ninety-day washout, crossover." That's a mouthful, but it explains exactly what was done, and how it was done.

Just how certain are you of the results? In statistical analysis, we employ what are known as "confidence intervals." A confidence interval is a figure that shows how certain we are that the results obtained lie within some range of scores. Incidentally, the research precedent that has been established for decades for preparing an article for journal publication is what determines the confidence intervals. For example, in physical sciences, the confidence interval is 99 percent. This means that if we plotted, in the experiment given above, each and every score (percent body fat) for every subject in the experiment, we would get a graph with a lot of dots on it, each dot representing one score. Assume that we see that the scores all fall within some range of scores—such as a low of 7.8 percent body-fat decrease and a high of 12.2 percent body-fat decrease. A 99 percent confidence interval states that, should this experiment be performed again—by anybody—the results of 99 of 100 scores (for each group) should fall within the range of scores between 7.8 percent body-fat decrease and 12.2 percent body-fat decrease.

The importance of anybody performing the same experiment, conducted exactly the same way, and getting the same results is what is known as "replication," and cannot be understated. This means that, if someone got significantly different results—say the average percent body-fat reduction was only 3.2 percent and the scores were in the range of 0.1 percent to 25.3 percent—something in the experiment is wrong, either in the initial experiment or in the one attempting to replicate it. This inability to replicate was obvious when, several years ago, some scientists claimed they had been able to create cold fusion—and in a sink in the home of one of the scientists, in Salt Lake City. When they published the results of their experiment, no one was able to replicate the study and get anywhere near the same results, so the claims of the original experimenters could not be believed.

Some additional points about scientific experiments need to be made. A person does not have to believe what a given researcher claims. All that person need do is repeat the experiment and compare results. In fact, most experiments are repeated many times, most often as a part of a larger experiment.

It is difficult for a consumer to know if a study and the results obtained are legitimate or not. I believe any consumer should be suspicious of any study that has not appeared in a peer-reviewed journal. I would also be suspicious of any study whose authors agreed that the publication decision would be up to the company funding the study. So, how might the manufacturers use results of their own studies, or ones they funded and were performed by someone else?

What they often do is use the experiment as the basis for their claims. For example, if the experiment I presented to you did show that one subject did experience a 12.2 percent reduction in percent body fat, the manufacturer will create an ad something like, "You can lose up to 12 percent body fat in just ninety days, just by taking our (name of product)." Is that statement true as far as it goes? Yes. Are the results, spread across the general population, likely? No, they are not. In fact, by the hypothetical experiment I presented to you, the odds are only 1 in 200 (only one subject in the entire study groups of two hundred had that high of percent body-fat reduction).

A manufacturer might use words such as: "A recent study at a major university showed that (some results)." Does the ad say when and where that study was done? Does the ad tell you where to write or call to get a copy of the study? And even if you found out where to locate the study, could you read and understand it?

When an experiment is completed and published in a refereed journal, it can be a bit difficult to read. Most experiments contain advanced statistical methodology and a lot of scientific jargon. If you do try to read one of these studies you'll see a pretty standard format. At the very beginning of the article there will be something called an "abstract," which is usually a fairly short one- or two-paragraph summary of what the experiment was designed to accomplish and how it was constructed. The content of the article then follows. At the end of the article is the summary or conclusion. These latter items state whether what was attempted (as stated in the abstract) was, in fact, accomplished and any recommendations for further research based upon the findings of the experiment.

In practice, the running of scientific experiments is both expensive and time-consuming.

All this is additional evidence that the manufacturer does not, or cannot, spend the resources to do studies to verify its claims. The hucksters find it far easier to simply hit you with lies and misrepresentations. Now you know what they know, and perhaps even more.

Ethics drives much of the experimentation. It is considered unethical to perform any experiment that could prove harmful to human participants. Most universities and medical centers have committees—usually called "IRBs," which means Institutional Review Boards—who will refuse to allow an experiment if they think harm might come to a participant. To get around this, scientists use animals—especially mice, dogs, and monkeys—whose physiology very closely approximates that of the human species.

When the experiment is completed it will have proven the hypothesis to be entirely true, entirely false, or limited as to truth. Also be aware that most of what is studied in the health and fitness industry affects the human body at the level of the individual cells. Most of the effects will be seen as a result of what occurs during digestion and because of your metabolism.

These two terms are poorly understood by the general public and need to be clearly explained. They tie back into the scientific method because everyone's metabolism is different, as is their individual digestive process, so results can vary because of them. Most hucksters never tell you that. This is incredibly subtle. The ad may contain the phrase, usually in very small print, "Individual results may vary." This tells you only *what* might vary (the results). It does not tell you *why* there might be variations (differences in each person's metabolism and digestion).

The implication is that people are different, so results might vary. That seems harmless enough. In point of fact, individual results might vary because of individual variances in digestion and metabolism. You might get no results if, say, you have a high metabolic rate which negates the action of the product, but you are not told this. See how you can get duped in a situation like that?

Thus, it's extremely helpful for you to know what metabolism is and how digestion works. What you are about to learn is how vitamins, minerals, herbs, and ergogenic supplements—whether taken in raw form or as part of what you eat and drink—are absorbed and utilized by your body. Again, be aware of how this is directly related to the scientific method and how differences in each individual may cause different results. Almost everything that is attempted to be proven in some way is a result of the impact on your metabolism and through digestion. When you understand these points you will have taken another major step toward becoming a formidable opponent of the hucksters.

Metabolism is the sum total of all the physical and chemical changes that take place in your body and, at the level of the individual cells within your body, all the material and energy transformations that occur. These material changes include every change that your body undergoes during all periods of your life—growth, maturity, and senescence (growing old). The energy changes include every change caused by food and drink that produces chemical energy and which is converted to mechanical energy or heat. All the energy in the body exists as potential (stored/inactive) or kinetic (in motion) energy. Chemical energy is stored in the bondings of chemical substances. When released, it becomes kinetic energy. Mechanical energy is directly involved in moving matter.

The material and chemical changes involve two fundamental processes: anabolism (building-up processes) and catabolism (tearing-down processes). Don't think tearing down means total destruction. It really means separating a substance into various, smaller components from which it is made.

Anabolism* is the conversion of what we eat and drink into constituents of protoplasm, a big word that simply means something that consists of inorganic (having no carbon molecule in them) substances, like water and mineral compounds, and organic (having carbon molecules) substances like proteins, carbohydrates, and fats. If you separated these organic substances and took a look at what they are made of, you'd find them to be 99 percent composed of carbon, oxygen, nitrogen, calcium, and phosphorus (very similar to the "building of the human body" diagram in chapter 1 at the lowest level—that of atoms). That remaining 1 percent is composed of potassium, sulfur, chlorine, sodium, magnesium, iron, copper, cobalt, manganese, zinc, and several others. Take a look at them. Don't they look suspiciously like the listed contents on the label of a vitamin/mineral supplement bottle? They should. That's *exactly* what they are!

In catabolism, larger substances are broken down into smaller and smaller substances. The terms of size—larger and smaller—may be confusing. It's just as accurate to think of more complex substances being broken down into simpler (less complex) substances. When you have broken down a substance into its most basic elements—called "end products"—the end products are secreted out of your body. Along the way, most substances are utilized by your body and I don't mean to imply that every substance simply keeps getting broken down into less complex substances—all of which wind up being secreted. That's not what happens. Some substances (compounds) never get broken down to the end-product stage.

---

*If you looked at the word anabolism and thought, *Hey. That word's awfully close to "anabolic," like in "anabolic steroids." Are those terms related?* Of course they are. Now you've got a better idea that anabolic steroids are something that builds up something else.

What does happen is that all this change comes about because of enzymes which are produced by your cells but act independent of them. Their whole purpose is to cause chemical changes in other substances without being changed themselves.

I've presented metabolism in the broad concept. To specifics: Each of the substances—like protein, carbohydrates, vitamins, minerals, etc.—all have their *own* metabolism; for example, protein metabolism or vitamin metabolism. The enzymes cause the building up or tearing down to occur in each and every type of metabolism.

In addition, I said enzymes are capable of acting independent of the cells. If you ask, "Well, where are they located?" the answer is, for example, in your saliva and digestive juices. They break down food and drink into their simpler compounds.

Just like the building of an organism as illustrated in chapter 1, a food—like a pizza—is nothing more than a process of continual combination of smaller elements into larger elements until the components of the pizza are identifiable, such as the bread (crust), tomato sauce, cheese, mushrooms, sausage, and the like (pick your own style). When you eat the pizza, the enzymes break the components into smaller and smaller elements that the body can utilize (absorb) or excrete. This utilization is caused by digestion. It occurs in the gastrointestinal tract (also called the GI tract) and what are called accessory digestive organs (tongue, teeth, salivary glands, gallbladder, liver, and pancreas). Most people think, incorrectly, that digestion takes place only in your stomach. Not true. The stomach breaks food particles down to compounds that the intestines can allow to absorb into the bloodstream.

Digestion is the chemical or mechanical process of breaking down what we eat and drink into substances that can be absorbed by the body. Point: Digestion is a part of your metabolism, not the other way around. I will use common terms to describe the process of digestion. I'll use a piece of steak to illustrate the food.

Digestion involves six activities. The activities are:

1. Ingestion;
2. Mechanical digestion;
3. Propulsion;

4. Chemical digestion;
5. Absorption;
6. Defecation.

Ingestion is simply putting the piece of steak into your mouth. Your mouth is the starting point of your digestive tract.

Mechanical digestion is the chewing of the steak, mixing it with the saliva (using your tongue), and, combined with propulsion, the churning and mixing of the food in your stomach so as to move it through your intestines.

Propulsion is simply the moving of the piece of steak from your mouth (starting point) to, ultimately, your anus for defecation (the ending point). Interestingly, from the time you swallow that piece of steak you have just chewed, its movement is caused entirely by reflex. The alternate waves of contraction and relaxation of the muscles in your digestive tract keep it moving. Think of this contraction and relaxation like taking a very long tube of toothpaste, with openings at both ends, and squeezing the tube at the top (its neck). Then, continue to simply go hand-over-hand, squeezing as you go, until you get to the end of the tube, moving the contents of the tube with each squeeze. In your body a mucus is secreted along the entire length of your digestive tract to protect the linings of the walls of the organs through which the meat is passing as well as to lubricate those walls and ease the movement of the meat. The propulsion is so effective, you could swallow the meat while standing and then immediately hang upside down and the meat would still continue to move "down" your digestive tract. This illustrates that digestion is not dependent upon gravity.

Chemical digestion is the breaking down of the meat into its chemical building blocks. This is where the enzymes enter the picture. It begins in your mouth, but for all practical purposes really kicks into high gear in your stomach and continues through your stomach into your small intestine, with some food residue being chemically digested in your large intestine. Be aware that the body absorbs the components of food at very different speeds. For example, the water in the meat is absorbed almost instantly; the carbohydrates are slower; the proteins even slower; and the fats slower yet.

Absorption is the process where the digested end products are transported throughout the body to the places they are to be utilized. This starts in your small intestine, after the food has been processed in, and moved out of, your stomach. These digested end products are carried by your blood vessels and lymph vessels to the various parts of your body. It's also here where the associated digestive organs come into play. The liver, pancreas, and gallbladder are all associated with the small intestine in this process.

The liver is a key organ. It's in the liver where nutrients passing through in the blood are picked up and processed yet further, or stored. For example, the fat-soluble vitamins A, D, E, and K are stored in the liver. It is also in the liver where detoxification occurs. One of three metabolic functions of the liver is to build amino acids into plasma proteins, perform transanimation to form nonessential amino acids, and convert the ammonia from their deanimation to urea, a less toxic excretory product.

Last, all the elements of that piece of meat have either been digested and sent on their way to be utilized by various parts of the body, or not digested. The *undigested* substances in the meat are propelled down the "tubes" of the small intestine to the large intestine (where what we describe as feces are formed) and then to the anus for defecation.

What the hucksters like to do is use statements such as "increase your metabolism," "aids in your digestion," "helps the body absorb the nutrients," and other similar claims. Nowhere is it stated in the ad how much (the quantitative amount) is the "increase," "aid," or "help." It's not stated because the amount is so small as to be ineffective in the ad—it won't get you excited so you'll spend your money—or it's simply not known.

VIPS

Most health and fitness ads cannot be substantiated by proof via the scientific method because they don't exist.

The scientific method is the only, singular, universally accepted method of proving whether a statement is univer-

sally true, universally false, or true within very limited circumstances and with limited applications.

If a scientific experiment has been correctly performed by accepted protocols, anybody, anywhere, should be able to perform the same experiment and get the same results every single time.

You, the taxpayers, fund most scientific studies. The results belong to you.

Hucksters will dupe you by taking scientific study results out of context or manipulate them to serve their own bias. They are aided and abetted by the media.

Metabolism and digestion are very specific processes. The hucksters use these terms in very general contexts, which result in these processes being associated with generalities that are misleading if not outright lies.

In the next chapter you will be able to actually measure the claims made by the hucksters. You will also learn that you can't measure the promised results when they are qualitative, not quantitative.

3

HOW *YOU* CAN MEASURE THE CLAIMS *AND* THE RESULTS
The Quantitative versus the Qualitative

What if an ad said: "You *will* increase your energy level *at least* 30 percent in thirty days"? Would you buy a product that made that claim? I think most of you probably would. I wouldn't, and here's why.

Suppose a second ad said: "You *can* increase your energy level *up to* 30 percent in thirty days." Note that the word "will" in the first ad (previous chapter) has been changed to "can," and the phrase "at least" has been changed to "up to."

This second ad is much less specific and certain as to the outcome (you *will* versus you *can*) and the amount of energy has been changed from a *minimum* of 30 percent in the first ad to a *maximum* of 30 percent in the second ad. Would you still want to spend your money on this second product? I doubt it, but unless you're aware of the subtle difference in the wording, you may not pay attention before you reach for your wallet, checkbook, or credit card.

"Increase energy." That's it. That's the whole claim. It should be obvious that in this ad there is absolutely nothing certain as to amount of that energy increase and there is no time frame stated. Save your money.

Even though the first ad seemed pretty straightforward it is, in fact, extremely subtle and has two big flaws. The subtlety is the fact that no starting point is mentioned. It is implied that it is the day before you begin taking the product for thirty days. You may think I'm splitting hairs on this one, but bear with me. The first flaw is that the manufacturer has no idea what your current energy level is. Do you? I really doubt it. How can you measure a 30 percent increase in something if you don't know the specific, "base" (or beginning) amount that will be increased 30 percent? You can't. The second flaw is that there is no indication *how* you are to measure the increase.

Now you're trapped. That first ad initially appeared as a pretty clear-cut *quantitative* statement, but it is really a sneaky *qualitative* statement.

Learn this point and learn it well: *If you cannot quantitatively measure the claim or the results of an ad, do not spend your money on that product.*

As a specific starting point, I am selecting energy (and lack thereof) because it is one of the most common complaints of patients to their physicians and, not accidentally, one of the most common claims that the manufacturers state that their product can improve or increase.

What you want is proof of the claim and/or the result. The proof has two steps. Step one is to define what it is you want to measure. This can be trickier than it seems. Define energy. Go ahead. It shouldn't be hard. After all, we've got a Department of Energy, utility companies that supply energy, countless ads that scream any number of phrases that include the word "energy," and we've even got a bunny that tools around our TV screens thumping on a drum. With all that exposure, energy should be easy to define, right? Just close your eyes and define energy.

I'm guessing that most of you either did not even try it or, if you did, you found it much harder than you thought it would be. In fact, probably very few of you know the definition of energy. That's one of the factors that ad makers count on—your ignorance.

Energy is simply defined as "the ability to do work." "Ability" means the same thing as "potential." Energy is measured in units called kilocalories. One kilocalorie is the amount of heat required to raise the temperature of one kilogram of water one degree Centigrade from 15 to 16 degrees or the amount of heat required to raise the temperature of about one quart of water from 59 to 60.8 degrees Fahrenheit.

When we are talking about exercise metabolism and human nutrition, we use the word "kilocalorie." It is represented by the capital letter "C." Capital C is also the Roman numeral for the quantity 100. It can get confusing if the "C" is used in the same sentence to mean degrees Centigrade as well as kilocalories. "Kilo" is a Greek prefix word that means 1,000. I'm presenting this because if you do read scientific literature (and a lot of texts used in schools), the metric notations are used instead of the familiar terms like one pound, one calorie, degrees Fahrenheit, etc. A small letter "c" (calorie) refers to the amount of heat needed to change one gram (about the size of two raindrops) of water from 15 to 16 degrees C (59 to 60.8 degrees F). To make my discussion simple for you, I will use the word "calorie"—without the kilo prefix. So just think of the familiar use of the word and you shouldn't get confused.

This ability to do work can be found in the chemical energy in the foods we eat and in the cells of the tissues of our bodies. Work is simply a force moving something against resistance. Blinking your eyes is work. Scratching your nose is work. Breathing is work. Lifting weights is work. Digesting food is work. Everything that is work expends energy; i.e., it "burns calories."

Here are the key points so far: If you move, you expend energy, measured in calories. You have some potential energy—the ability to do work—already in your cells and when you eat you take in more potential energy that contains calories.

All the major classes of organic nutrients contain calories:

- Protein has four calories per gram;
- Carbohydrate has four calories per gram;
- Fat has nine calories per gram.

One gram is 0.03215 ounces. One pound of fat contains very nearly 3,500 calories.

Here's where it all starts to come together. To free this potential energy—in effect, to convert the *potential* for movement to *actual* movement—you need to transform this chemical energy in your body to mechanical energy or heat. This is exactly what metabolism is and this transformation occurs at the level of the cells in your body.

Bringing the ads back into all this, "increase energy" really has *two* meanings: either the *ability* to perform work or the *actual transformation* of potential energy into movement. Now that is quite subtle, if I do say so myself. But have you ever seen *any* ad by *any* body at *any* time state or even infer this? I doubt it. It all goes back to the use of words/phrases you don't know but think you do.

Now that we know a bit more about energy and the calories that supply it, I'm going to show you how to measure what your energy level is and how to measure any change over time.

Go lie down. Just lie there quietly. Since you're still alive, your basic metabolism is working. The amount of energy you are expending while you are at rest for one minute is equivalent to one MET. MET stands for "Metabolic Equivalent."

When you do things, your MET level rises to some *multiple* of your resting metabolic rate. For example, low-impact aerobics uses 5.0 METs; walking at a 2 mph pace on a firm, level surface uses 2.5 METs; competitive soccer uses 10.0 METs. Said another way, those METs of 5.0, 2.5, and 10.0 require 5, 2.5, and 10 times more energy than your body requires when it is at rest. If you want to know what almost every exercise/movement you can do uses in METs, buy or check out a terrific book, *ACSM's Resource Manual for Guidelines for Exercise Testing and Prescription.*[1]

To measure the amount of energy you use even more precisely than with METs, you can compute it by finding your VO_2, pronounced just as it appears, "vee-oh-two." VO_2 represents your use of oxygen (oxygen uptake). If you're lying on your bed and you get up, your heart starts to beat faster. This results in your taking in more oxygen because more oxygen is now required by your body. Your heart may pump more of this oxygenated blood around your cardiovascular system to: (1) deliver oxygen and nutrients to the cells so they can perform work, and (2) pick up the by-products, like carbon dioxide (CO_2) that you eventually exhale. The amount of blood that is pumped with each heartbeat—called your heart's stroke volume—will also increase.

If an ad says, "Increase your energy," how do you *know* if the product being advertised works? Simple. Compute your energy before and after taking the product. What follows are the formulas for computing the amount of energy you use for various exercises that most of us can do. They are taken from another terrific book, *Metabolic Calculations—Simplified*, by Dr. David P. Swain and Dr. Brian C. Leutholtz.[2] The good doctors have removed all the metric terminology and equations and converted them into something even I can understand.

Here are the formulas that should interest you:

WALKING:

VO_2 = 3.5 + 2.68(speed in mph) + 0.48(speed in mph)(% grade).

The "% grade" is a *whole number*, so if you're walking up, say a 6% grade, you would enter "6" in the formula and *not* 0.06. If the surface is flat, enter zero for % grade.

RUNNING—on a treadmill:

VO_2 = 3.5 + 5.36(speed in mph) + 0.24(speed in mph)(% grade).

RUNNING—outdoors:

VO_2 = 3.5 + 5.36(speed in mph) + 0.48(speed in mph)(% grade). (you can use a protractor to sight the % grade.)

BENCH or STAIR STEPPING:

VO_2 = 0.35(rate) + 0.061(rate)(height in inches).

The "rate" is the number of steps per minute. A "step" occurs when you have completed a "cycle," which means for example, that if you're standing flat on the floor, then you step up with one foot and then the other onto the bench (or stair or box) and then step back down, one foot at a time onto the floor, that "up-up-down-down cycle" counts as *one* step.

Here's an example using the walking equation. Assume you're walking on a flat surface (no grade at all) at a pace of 3 miles per hour. What is your VO_2?

Just fill in the numbers and be careful as you make the calculation!

VO_2 = 3.5 + 2.68(speed in mph) + 0.48(speed in mph)(% grade)
VO_2 = 3.5 + 2.68(3) + 0.48(3)(0)
VO_2 = 3.5 + 8.04 + 0.48(0)

$$VO_2 = 3.5 + 8.04 + 0$$
$$VO_2 = 11.54^*$$

If you wanted to test a claim made of "more energy," you can use an allowable variation of the scientific method. You become an experimental group of one. Here's what I mean. First, measure your VO_2. Then consume whatever it is you've purchased for thirty days. Do *nothing different* at all in your life *except* consuming that product. At the end of thirty days, measure your VO_2 again. Tip: Take each measurement at the same time of the day, and the same time after you've consumed the meal nearest the time when you take the measurements.

If the VO_2 is larger the second time you took it, you have scientific proof that your energy has *increased* and the product was the cause! I'm using thirty days for a reason. Whenever you do something different to your body—like exercising, taking supplements, etc.—the greatest changes occur *earliest* in your "program." Thirty days is enough time to make a measurable difference, if there is going to be one.

You may want to go back and read the previous paragraph again. It is a stunning disclosure of proof as to a claim and the claimed results.

I know someone out there is saying, "Wait a minute. How can I measure my speed so I can include it in the formula?" There are numerous ways, but some of the most common are to use a treadmill at a health club; buy a pedometer that has the mph readout on it (don't pay more than twenty dollars for one of these or you're paying too much); take any measured distance and time yourself and convert to miles per hour. For example, a football field is 100 yards long. If you walk from goal line to goal line in one minute, your walking speed is 3.41 mph. Here's the proof: There are 1,760 yards in a mile. Divide the 1,760 by the 100 and you get 17.6. This means you'd walk a mile in 17.6 minutes. Divide 60 minutes by 17.6 to get 3.41 mph. Whatever you do—walk, run, or step—continue that movement for at least five minutes to get a more useful time frame of energy expenditure.

---

*Where people make a mistake is in the last component of the equation. The grade is *zero*, but many people will multiply the 0.48 times the speed in mph, and then leave out the multiplier—zero—and come up with some number *other* than zero. Remember the correct rule: *Any number multiplied by zero gives you an answer of zero.*

How would you like to know how many calories you burn up each minute? Take the answer from the equation for your VO_2 we used on page 72—in this case it was 11.54. Then find the answers in the following equations. Unfortunately, you'll have to use some metric figures, but I'll convert them for you.

The first answer you'll need to find is the number of liters (L) per minute of oxygen you use. Let's say you weigh 220 pounds. There are 2.2 pounds in one kilogram, so divide 220 by 2.2 to get a body weight of 100 kilograms. You'll also substitute the answer from above, 11.54 for VO_2. That formula is:

VO_2 in L per minute $= VO_2 \times$ (body weight in kilograms/1000)
VO_2 in L per minute $= 11.54 \times (100/1000)$
VO_2 in L per minute $= 11.54 \times (1/10)$
VO_2 in L per minute $= 1.54$
Calories used per minute $= VO_2$ in L per minute $\times 5$
Calories burned per minute $= 1.54 \times 5$
Calories burned per minute $= 7.70$

If you want to play a few games here, you could say, "Okay, if I walked at 3 mph on a flat surface, how many calories would I burn up in thirty minutes?" Just multiply the answer you just computed, above—7.70—times 30. Answer: *231 calories*.

If you wanted to know how long it would take you to burn off one pound of fat (recall there are 3,500 calories in one pound of fat), just divide 3,500 by 7.70. Answer: *454 minutes* (a little over 7.5 hours).

You may be saying, "You mean to tell me I have to walk for seven and a half hours to lose a pound of fat?" That's exactly correct, but consider that if you only walked 30 minutes a day, in one year you'd lose 24.09 pounds of fat (multiply 365 days times 30 minutes times 7.70 calories, and then divide that product of those three multiplications by 3,500) and you're not straining yourself to do it.

You'll see a lot more about weight loss, METs, etc. in chapter 12.

What you have just been given is the method to prove whether or not a product that claims to increase your energy does in fact do so—even when the manufacturer has no idea either how much energy you have before you start taking that product or what kind of exercise you will be doing.

You may be thinking, *This is all well and good, but how can I figure my energy expenditure (VO$_2$) if I want to do something other than walk, jog, or step up and down?* Good question. Easy answer. Just get a copy of the *ACSM Resource Manual*, find the METs for whatever exercises you want, and *multiply* that figure by 3.5. Example: I looked at raking the lawn in their tables. The number of METs for raking the lawn is 4.0. The VO$_2$ is simply 4.0 times 3.5, for an answer of *14.0*.

If you want to find the METs, just *divide* the VO$_2$ by 3.5. In the walking example above, the VO$_2$ of 11.54 can now be divided by 3.5 to give that walking exercise a MET of *3.297*. Said another way, that walking exercise requires 3.297 times more energy than quietly resting.

Manufacturers will hate you for what you have just learned. You can take almost any type of movement/exercise and compute not only how much change in energy, if any, results and even the number of calories you have burned.

I know this explanation of energy has been lengthy, at least by ad standards with their insipid, abbreviated claims. But don't you think the ad makers could come up with something a little more specifically quantitative and/or a little more informative? Or maybe they think you're just too dumb to understand it. I don't.

Because you are learning tricks and tools of the enemy, let's have some more fun and take a shot at measuring some of the following phrases, taken from actual ads, such as "less fat," "increased metabolism," "add tone," "feel younger," "lose pounds," "restore youth," and "breathe easier."

First, notice that none of these phrases has any time frame attached to them. None tells you *how fast* the product is supposed to work. That alone should cause you to slap the "**REJECT**" stamp on them.

Second, there is no definite, quantifiable amount of change attached to any of them. Lay the "**REJECT**" on them one more time.

Third, take each phrase individually and determine if something there can be measured. (A correctly worded ad should say: "If you take our product for ninety days, make no change in your diet or exercise level, you will lose between two to six pounds.") "Lose fat" is a phrase that can be measured in a quantifiable way. In fact, I have measured patients four different ways. The first and *least* precise is by computing the Body Mass Index (BMI). BMI is the ratio of weight to height in adults and gives you body composition; i.e., degree of fat in the body (the level of obesity). There are 2.2 pounds in a kilogram and 39.37 inches in a meter. Assume you're five feet, ten inches tall and weigh 160 pounds. What's your BMI? Divide 160 by 2.2 and you get your body weight in kilograms—72.73. You're 70 inches tall, so divide 70 by 39.37 to get your height in meters—1.78. The formula for BMI is:

BMI = weight in kilograms/height in meters squared
BMI = 72.73/1.78 squared
BMI = 72.73/3.168
BMI = *22.96*

According to the American College of Sports Medicine and the American College of Cardiologists, any BMI score below 25 is indicative of very low body fat. A score of 25.0–29.9 is Grade I obesity, and any BMI above 27 indicates definite obesity. Scores of 30–40 are severe obesity and above 40 you have extreme obesity.

The second method is the most reliable but also the most expensive. It is called "hydrostatic weighing." It requires you to *exhale* and *then* go under water in a small tank of water. You read that correctly. Most people, if they have to submerge themselves under water want to inhale first. Not with hydrostatic weighing. That extra air you want to inhale gives added buoyancy to the body and results in a computation that is incorrectly lower as to the amount of fat in a person's body.

The third method is via bioelectrical impedance analysis (BIA). This is the best compromise between cost and accuracy. In this method a little wrap is placed around a toe or finger and a harmless 50kHz current is passed through the body at that point. It's quick, painless, noninvasive, given with the greatest privacy (no disrobing), and it's easy to administer. BIA measures the difference in resistance to electrical current in lean body mass and body fat mass. Lean body mass has a greater amount of water than body fat, so the higher the water content, the better the conductance (less impedance).

The last method is the skinfold test in which a skinfold caliper is placed on various positions of the body. The caliper looks like a large pincer (about eight inches long), but it is neither sharp nor painful. I strongly recommend that measurements be taken in at least five different places on the body. This is a very inexpensive method to determine body fat; however, not many people are skilled at it. I also strongly suggest you look at the *ACSM Resource Manual* (pp. 95-97) and see how it should be done. I once employed a person to take skinfold measurements for my patients. I came to find out he told the interviewer he had given " . . . over five hundred skinfold caliper tests to people." When I observed, I found that was probably true—but they were all given *incorrectly*. Look especially for the exact positioning of the caliper, the amount of skin pinched, and the time the caliper enfolds the skin.

Regardless of which method you use, use the same method every time you are tested. Have the measurements taken at least thirty days apart. Just as with energy measurements, you want to test, give yourself thirty days to take the product/do the exercise, and then test again and notice any change in the answers.

"Increased metabolism" cannot be measured in this case because these words do not specify which metabolism is being increased. Again, there is an overall metabolism for your entire body called the organism's metabolism or "whole body" metabolism. There is also protein metabolism, carbohydrate metabolism, fat metabolism, vitamin metabolism, amino acid metabolism, etc. Do not—repeat—do not get suckered into assuming which metabolism the ad refers to, for if you do, you again are completing the implication made by the manufacturer and this only leads to you being duped yet again and wasting your money. It's the manufacturer's responsibility to tell you which metabolism is being referenced.

Some manufacturer may throw a tantrum and say, "I'm talking about whole body metabolism!" Why didn't you state that clearly in your ad? If that ever happens, ask to see the results of the direct calorimetry stud(y/ies). The manufacturer won't know what to say. Know why? You can measure whole body metabolism by direct calorimetry. In fact, it's the most precise way to do it. Unfortunately, to perform direct calorimetry requires the study subject to be placed in an airtight room where heat is released, the temperature inside the chamber rises, and a circulating jacket of water transfers the heat to the environment. Direct calorimetry is very, very expensive. Best bet is that the manufacturer never had the direct calorimetry study(ies) done, so they can't produce any test results. Of course, even if the results were made available to you, you know enough about the scientific method to determine if the study was done according to the strict protocols required and whether they have been published in refereed, scientific journals. The manufacturer relies on the hope that no one will question what "increased metabolism" means but will be influenced by the implication that such an increase will mean weight loss.

"Add tone" usually conjures up pictures of muscular, tanned people supposedly the epitome of health. Here we go with the implications again but the wheels really come off the wagon when you define the word "tone." According to *Taber's Cyclopedic Medical Dictionary*, it says, "tone. 1. That state of a body or any of its organs or parts in which the functions are healthy and normal."[3] I ask you, how in the world can you add tone to a body? Tone is not a substance. It is a state (or condition). It's like being happy. How do you "add happy"? If you *add* tone, by definition you're adding something normal to something normal. Normal plus normal equals normal. Tone is not something you ingest into your body. Good grief, how dumb do the hucksters think we are? I think they think we are incredibly dumb.

"Feel younger" is much like "add tone." "Younger" is an indefinite amount. Does it mean ten minutes? Six weeks? Ten years? The ad is silent as to that answer. You may get subtly duped into trying to differentiate or relate "younger" with "more energy," since most of us would say, "I had more energy when I was younger." If you do that, you've really twisted yourself into a knot because, if you didn't measure your level of energy some time in the past, you have no quantitative basis with which to compare it today. So, what you wind up doing is differentiating or comparing one indefinite—"more energy"—with another indefinite—"feel younger." The differentiation or comparison must logically fall flat on its face.

"Lose pounds" has possibilities. Not many, but a few. First, the ad does not state how fast you will begin losing pounds and for how long.

It does not state how many pounds will be lost. It also does not tell you how many pounds of *what*. This is important. If you lose just water, you could be in real trouble. A 6 percent decrease in body weight solely from water, without replacement, and you will suffer serious decreases in muscular strength and endurance. Lose more than 10 percent without replacement and you are history (as in d-e-a-d).

You can measure a loss of pounds. Just hop on a scale. Measure your abdomen with a tape measure. But why buy any product that is so indefinite as to the claim? The answer is the same as the opening words of the first chapter; because you hear what you want to hear and see what you want to see. And you get duped. And you waste money. And you get frustrated. And you get embarrassed. And you get angry. Follow my advice and this won't happen to you.

"Restore youth" is "feel younger"'s cousin. Restore has a more permanent implication to it. A feel can be fleeting, but restore, why, we're talking the big leagues here. In fact, I dedicate the whole of chapter 13 to this topic. I think you will be surprised.

"Breathe easier" should look familiar. It is. It's part of the headline of an ad illustrated in the previous chapter (page 52). "Breathe easier" has three anatomical and physiological possibilities, but you're not told which one. The first is your nose. "Breathe easier" would imply the removal of some restriction to breathing through your nose. The second is your trachea (windpipe) and your lungs. There is the same implication here as for the nasal passages. The third possibility is a combination of the first and second possibilities.

You can't do much to quantitatively measure your inhaling and exhaling (one of each constitutes one respiration) relative to your nose. Of course, if you're an athlete like me who stuck his nose in front of too many opponents and have a deviated septum (a broken nose with cartilage blocking air passage in a nostril), no drug or pill or plant is going to remove the obstruction. Surgery is the only option.

Your lungs and windpipe are another matter. The amount of air exhaled can easily be measured by what is called a "spirometer." There's nothing magical about it. It's just a box with a few dials/gauges on its face, a tube coming out of it, and a disposable mouthpiece through which you exhale. As you exhale, the air goes down the tube, into the box and into a bellows (just an inflatable bladder).

The air exhaled is measured and displayed on a tape or screen on the spirometer. You can get two essential measurements.

The first is FEV_1—which means Forced Expiratory Volume in One Second. This is how much air you can "explosively" exhale in one second. The second measurement is called the FVC—which means Forced Vital Capacity. It is the total amount of air you can exhale for as long as you are continually exhaling. Most physicians' offices, hospitals, outpatient clinics, and many health clubs have them. The tests shouldn't cost more than twenty-five dollars.

The essential point is that if you can "breathe easier" you should be able to inhale and exhale (respire) with less effort than before you began to take some product or prescription. If that's the case—and it should be—at least some obstruction(s) should have been removed from your air passages and the lining of your lungs should have more elasticity than before the "treatment." That should result in higher numbers being attained on the FEV_1 and the FVC tests. No other result is possible. The hucksters are betting that you won't take the trouble to have them done. They are betting that you will base your "better breathing" on a mere subjective evaluation of "before" and "after."

What follows at this point may seem to be more logically placed in the previous chapter; it really is not. What happens if you read or hear of a study and the results you measure for yourself are not even close to those in the study? This happens more often than you think. What you should do if this occurs is look for what we call a "meta-analysis." This is simply a study of a whole bunch of related studies. Think of it as a "summary study." Rather than try and slog through fifty studies on the effect of a particular product on your muscle metabolism, it's a lot easier to just read one study that combines (summarizes) the results of those fifty studies. The easiest way to find such a study is to call a university or medical school library and let the research librarians do the work for you. If they find something, they will usually fax or mail you the meta-analysis. Mailing is usually fifteen cents a page for photocopying—plus postage—and faxing is usually a dollar a page.

In closing, it should be obvious that this representative sample of ad words and phrases clearly shows that most are meaningless. Those that contain possibilities as to quantitative measurement are most likely not backed by true scientific studies. *The whole question is not whether something works at all, but whether it works as advertised.* Since the ads are often indefinite and misleading, how can anybody know when the manufacturers will wake up and put truth, the whole truth, and nothing but the truth in their ads? All the manufacturer wants you to do is complete the implication—that you'll get the maximum stated or inferred benefits from the product—and spend your money.

VIPS

Any ad that contains qualitative (indefinite) words or phrases is meaningless.

If you can't quantitatively measure the claim or results of an ad, don't buy that product.

You can measure your energy expenditure and calories burned. This is done the way you need it—quantitatively.

Pay no attention to an ad that uses words or phrases that don't fit accepted medical, scientific, or legitimate dictionary definitions. If you don't know, look in the appropriate dictionary.

For the rest of the book, the topics are very product-specific. The next chapter is all about vitamins—the biggest moneymaker for the health and fitness industry. It's also where you waste most of your money. Turn the page and find out how they do it and how to avoid it.

NOTES

1. American College of Sports Medicine, *ACSM's Resource Manual for Guidelines for Exercise Testing and Prescription*, 3d ed. (Baltimore: William & Wilkins, 1998), see especially pp. 657–65.

2. David P. Swain and Brian C. Leutholtz, *Metabolic Calculations—Simplified* (Baltimore: William & Wilkins, 1997).

3. Clayton L. Thomas, ed., *Taber's Cyclopedic Medical Dictionary* (Philadelphia: F. A. Davis Company, 1993), p. 2005.

4

VITAMINS
The Good, the Bad, and the Expensive

The vitamin hucksters have become extremely skilled at taking something that is essentially simple, making it seem complex, and serving up gigantic helpings of this self-created misinformation for a price. Here's an essential point to burn into your brain: *All vitamins are chemicals. That's all they are.* Depending on their chemical structure, we can look at them and say, "That is vitamin A or C, or niacin (or whatever)." So, it does not matter if a vitamin is in its natural state in a food or beverage, has been added back into something after manufacture (like a cereal), or has been synthesized (manufactured) in some lab and put in a pill, *they are all the same!* Thus, since all vitamins are the same, it is the sales pitch—and not the product—that must "differentiate" the product in the mind of the potential consumer. The manufacturers know this, but they will never tell you. They want you to believe that their vitamin, or combinations of vitamins, is better, and will do more for you than a competitor's product. Hogwash. The prize they win when you are duped and thereby needlessly spend your money on vitamins is in the billions of dollars.

I saw an ad for a vitamin and mineral supplement named "Comprehensive Formula Nutrition," which aired on the Time-Warner cable channel 38, from 7 to 7:30 P.M., on 24 July 1999 in the Atlanta area. One of the people in that ad was the actress Marilu Henner, from the *Taxi* show. Let's look at some of her statements and see if you think she was trying to take the viewer for a ride. She stated, among other things that, ". . . vitamins give you a renewed sense of energy . . . reduce stress. . . . I found I had less stress at home. . . . I found my other vitamins were not being completely absorbed . . ." and ". . . a balanced and scientifically advanced formula. . . ."

First, vitamins do not give anybody a renewed sense of energy. I just explained energy—what it is and how it's measured—in some detail in the previous chapter. This idea of "renewed sense" is impossible, not only because of the measurement requirement (she makes it very nebulous and indefinite), but also because the word "sense" means a feeling or perception produced through the organs of touch, taste, etc., or resulting from a particular condition of some part of the body. And here's the kicker: *No vitamin contains any energy whatsoever*.

Some people will try to fool you and say, "Yeah, but vitamins release energy in the body." No, they do not. They *assist* in the release of energy—from fats, protein, and carbohydrate—and it's only the B-vitamins that do so, *and* the body automatically regulates the amount of energy released. *The amount of energy released is NOT increased by taking more vitamins*.

Second, there has never been a single, valid, scientific study that has proven that vitamins reduce stress. Period.

Third, when Ms. Henner says, ". . . I found I had less stress at home . . ." I can only wonder if she shot the plumber when she saw the bill. Did that reduce her stress? And was there more, the same, or less stress when at the job, in the commute, at the beauty parlor, etc.? And the ad never says when she "found" this less stress (before or after taking these vitamins?). And how long was this "less stress" experienced? And was the stress level she was experiencing "before" due to events that did/did not occur/changed or was it due to how she responded to those stressful situations? Obviously, the ad never addresses these sound bites and legitimate questions. In fact, she does not state which kind(s) of stress is being referred to—physical or emotional. According to the American Dietetic Association, it is an absolute fact that there is virtually no evidence that emotional stress causes a greater need for vitamins.

It is not true that a person who is recovering from major surgery, fracture, or burns needs extra vitamins. Since the ad presented no evidence as to the type of stress being addressed, we are left with the implication (there's that word again) that it is emotional stress to which Ms. Henner refers. And, even if her level of stress was reduced, was the result cause and effect or simply coincidence, vis-à-vis the vitamins?

☐ #8. THE PRINCIPLE OF PILFERAGE AND PROTECTION

The Principle of Pilferage and Protection is based upon two premises: First, that exercise, stress, or smoking somehow "robs" your body of essential vitamins or totally depletes your water-soluble vitamins on a *daily* basis, and (2) you must take vitamin supplements as a form of "insurance" against this supposed loss of vitamins. *Exercise, stress, and smoking do not rob your body of any vitamins. And, if you buy vitamin supplements because you believe they do, the only guarantee you will get is a guarantee that you're wasting your money.*

As to the fourth quote I presented from the ad—"I found my other vitamins were not being comletely absorbed"—I'm afraid this whole idea of absorption is not understood by the general public, which is the way the hucksters want to keep it. Read on, and in a very few minutes you will have that understanding.

Some manufacturers will even use the word "bioavailability" to mean absorption. They are not the same. In simple terms, as it relates to vitamins, absorption refers to the percent of the vitamin that either exits—unused—from the body, or passes through some surface of the body into its fluids and tissues to be stored or utilized. Scientifically, bioavailability has always referred to minerals, not vitamins. Here are some additional factoids about vitamins as they relate to absorption:

1. *No vitamin is totally absorbed by the body.* Said another way, *every* vitamin has an absorption rate of *less* then 100 percent.

2. The highest absorption rates of every vitamin occur when the vitamin is a *natural* part of the food ingested.
3. The second-highest absorption rate of every vitamin occurs when *synthetic* vitamins are ingested *with* meals.
4. The lowest absorption rate of every vitamin occurs when *synthetic* vitamins are ingested *between* meals.
5. Fat-soluble vitamins (A, D, E, and K) are absorbed more slowly in the body than water-soluble vitamins.
6. For a normal, healthy adult, the absorption takes an average of one to three hours.
7. All vitamins are stored in the body—even water-soluble vitamins—and it would take *several weeks* (yes, I said w-e-e-k-s) for the body to deplete its natural store of *any* vitamin to a potentially dangerous, low level, and that assumes *no intake whatsoever* of that vitamin during the weeks in question.
8. You may know what amounts of vitamins (and minerals) are in your body by a series of blood tests that costs $500 to $800, depending on the price structure of the blood lab that performs the analysis.

I would love to know how Ms. Henner discovered that her vitamins were not being totally absorbed. Again, we are left to ponder whether she was referring to another group of synthetic vitamins she had been taking; the fact that she just learned the eight points I presented above (and if that's the case, why is she buying/touting synthetic vitamins in the first place?); and how long before the ad was filmed did she discover this earth-shattering fact? It is also a fact that the body will excrete all of the water-soluble vitamins it doesn't need, so *of course* not all of the vitamins are absorbed *regardless* of what the absorption rate is.

Her last statement—"a balanced and scientifically advanced formula"—is as hollow and misleading as all the rest. "Balanced" could mean any figure—pick 15 percent, but any figure will do—of the adult, average daily requirements of all vitamins. That does fit a definition of "balanced," as none is any more or less prevalent than any other, but the ad doesn't say. It would be nice to know the actual amounts of each vitamin and mineral, especially as to what is recommended by the FDA, for example.

"Scientifically advanced formula" is absurd. The words don't tell you on which base the formula is advanced, how measured, or by how much. Scientists know what we need and in what amounts. There is nothing new, except how it is labeled, as will be explained below.

In summary, the ad was a classic case of a testimonial being used that was full of innuendo, inaccuracies, implications, and the not-so-subtle siren song, "Hey, everybody, this stuff did all these things for me and they can do the same for you!"

All vitamins are good, but too much or too little can be very bad for you. Also, synthesized vitamins are always more expensive than vitamins that are in the natural state in foods.

As I alluded to previously, if you consider nature to be a factory that produces vitamins, and compare that to what is produced (synthesized, as in synthetic vitamins) at a chemical company in which vitamins are produced, there is *no difference*. Remember how we built a human organism in chapter 2. Vitamin structure can be explained in just the first two steps of that illustration. Vitamins are simply atoms that are strung together to make the molecules that are identified as vitamins. There *is* one big difference—the price. Synthetic vitamins are more expensive than nature's product—all the time, every time, and with no exceptions.

Hucksters play this spin on price for all it's worth. The same ad that included Ms. Henner had this "fantastic" offer. The offer was for a thirty-day supply of the product. The "value" of that thirty-day supply was "normally" $29.95. However, as a "special introductory offer," you could get a thirty-day supply for only $9.95 PLUS a special newsletter (that was stated as being a "twenty-dollar value") *all* for $29.95. Let me rip this facade apart.

First of all, how could the "normal" price be $29.95 when it had never been on the market before? Please note, dear reader, that the ad said it was a "special *introductory* offer."

Second, it is obvious that the value of the newsletter was arbitrarily set. It is only valued as it is so that the "special cost" of the product—$9.95—can be added to some number (in this case the twenty bucks for the newsletter) so as to arrive at a market price of $29.95. Magically (well, not really), that $29.95 is *exactly* equal to the price of a thirty-day supply of the product if you had to pay retail (that is, sometime *after* this special *introductory* offer has expired).

Third, you think, *Where did the manufacturer come up with the $29.95 in the first place?* Hold that thought for a few minutes while I provide you with even more useful information.

Fourth, did you ever wonder why the containers of the supplements that you see advertised or displayed are many times larger than necessary to hold the contents? This is really subtle. You see, the actual ingredients are so small that you'd never buy them if you saw how small they are. So the manufacturers make great big bottles that are mostly filled with two things—air and cotton. They will try and tell you they couldn't list all the ingredients on the bottle if the bottle were smaller. Not so. If you look at the amount of space in the bottle that contains the tablets and then look at the quantity contained in the bottle as stated on the label (such as "30 tablets"), you've got to ask yourself, "Look, if this bottle is only 10 percent full of tablets, why can't the manufacturer just add ten times more tablets and make the bottle full?" Good question. The answer has everything to do with profit. Please hold onto *that* thought for a few minutes while I give you some more necessary information.

Fifth, haven't you ever wondered why a tablet that contains only *one* vitamin is so much *larger* than a *multi*vitamin supplement tablet, even though they *both* contain the *same amount* of that one vitamin? The reason is that the manufacturers want you to believe you are getting something "substantial" regarding the size of the tablet relative to its cost. So the majority of the actual "content" of the tablet is not the vitamin/supplements, but what is called "filler." Filler is essentially an inert substance that is used solely to make the tablet larger. Most, if not all, of the vitamin/multivitamin tablets contain *far more* filler than they do nutrient(s). To be very blunt about it, if you took the average daily requirement of all the vitamins and minerals a normal healthy adult in this country needs, made them into a pill with no filler, you could *far* more easily pick up that pill with a pair of tweezers than with your fingers.

Okay, you've been holding long enough. Now let's take a look at the profits. I called several managers with the largest Wall Street brokerage firms and asked them: "What is the markup in the vitamin/mineral industry?" They called their industry analysts who worked for these firms in New York. The markup is at least 400 percent! That's just for the contents. The packaging, transportation, and advertising is about one-third of the contents cost. What this means in raw numbers is that, if you had a bottle of vitamins with a retail price of $30, the cost of the contents is *not more* than $7.50. The packaging, transportation, and advertising would be—at most—another $2.50. So, the profit is *at least* $20 ($30 less $7.50 less $2.50)!

Note: The gentlemen said I could not use their names or that of the firms because they had to work continually with different industry executives and felt those executives would "clam up" if they felt their "inside info" was being given out to the public. They further added that their firms needed the legitimate information provided by these various executives to give to their firms and from which all kinds of information is made available to investors/potential investors. I see their point.

If you don't believe Wall Street analysts, try this on for size: It is a quote from Frank I. Katch and William D. McArdle's great book *Introduction to Nutrition, Exercise, and Health*.[1] On page 103 of the book, it is stated, "The average profit in a single dose of the RDA for *all* of the vitamins exceeds 1300%. If you doubt such excessive profit margins, the wholesale cost for the RDA of all the vitamins in a single capsule is less than one cent!"

☐ #9. THE PRINCIPLE OF THE BOOKEND BOOBY TRAP

The Principle of the Bookend Booby Trap works like this: The ad begins (one end) with some amazing claims. This is meant to grab your attention and move you emotionally and make you pay attention to the rest of the ad. It then proceeds to state a lot of other claims, all designed to convince you somewhere along the line that you just have to buy this product. At the conclusion of the ad (the other end of the bookend) the huckster refuses to let go of you. To make the last attempt at entrapment, the ad will present an offer that is supposedly just too good to pass up. The typical ones are something like:

- A special price reduction for a limited time only as an intro-ductory offer;
- Giving a multiple offer at the one price ("Buy two *now* and get one absolutely free!");
- A variation on the preceding tactic is to add—not the product itself in some multiple—but something else of value like a tape, a newsletter, etc.

Basically, it's a lot of cheap stuff to get you to buy under the feeling of "I can get all that for just that one, low price? Gimme the phone, Agnes, this is too good a deal to pass up!" Go to it, sucker . . .

I tried a trick on a person who answered the phone at the number I called for something I saw advertised on cable TV. The offer was for some car polish. The ad said that if I ordered right now, I could get two bottles for the price of one—$19.95. When I called I said, "Look, if one bottle is a $19.95 value, instead of sending me two bottles for $19.95, why don't you send me just one bottle—you keep the second bottle—and also send me a check for $19.95, the value of the second bottle?" The person on the other end hung up on me. You might try this with the ad that Ms. Henner was in. Tell the order taker you will pay $9.95 for the nutrients, but they can keep the twenty-dollar newsletter and to send you a check for the twenty dollars instead.

Don't let the hucksters drop guilt feelings on you. They may kick and scream because you are critical of their ads. You are *not* to be blamed for being cynical. *They* are the ones who scripted, revised, and edited the ads—not you. And when the ads are critically analyzed under the cold glare of scientific scrutiny, the majority of ads are shown to be outright lies and/or misleading and/or include misrepresentations.

*   *   *

Let me supply you with a few more important facts. I'll present them in the form of questions and then answer each one: (1) Just exactly what is it that vitamins *do*? (2) How do I know how much I have in my body (without paying $500 to $800)? (3) How much should be in my body? (4) How much is too much? (5) How little is too little?

The answer to the first question is that without any vitamins at all in your body you would die. They regulate the body's organism metabolism and all its other metabolisms; they assist in the release of energy within the body; and they figure importantly in the manufacture of body tissues. Vitamins do all of this at the cellular level.

The answer to the remaining four questions will be done collectively and requires a good sense of humor. This is so because we have to deal with the federal government, among other entities, and play a game of alphabet soup. To explain, let me begin with the federal government—specifically the Food and Drug Administration (FDA). It has no fewer than five acronyms that relate to nutrient intakes.

MDR

*M*inimum *D*aily *R*equirement. This is the amount *below* which a person could suffer various maladies. The MDR does not exist today, at least by that label. It was originally intended to be a set of statistical norms, but at a time when the determination of the norms was not possible (forty years ago). When science established the norms, the designation was dropped to avoid confusion.

USRDA

*U.S. R*ecommended *Daily A*llowance. This is the amount that Americans could, if they ingested on a daily basis, be sure of having no problems of acquiring any nutrient deficiencies. It does not mean one has to ingest *exactly* the amount stated in the USRDA; rather, it is acceptable for the vast majority of Americans. Note that the word "Daily" is italicized. The reason will be explained below.

DRV

*D*aily *R*eference *V*alues. This is the amount, based on a diet of 2,000 calories, that would provide what is recommended in the USRDA. If you are above or below 2,000 calories, you would adjust your nutrient intake by the same percentage.

RDI

*R*eference *D*aily *I*ntake. This is an amount based on the National Academy of Sciences' RDA of 1968. The RDA will be explained below.

DV

*D*aily *V*alue. The government, in its infinite wisdom, felt the DRV and RDI were too confusing, so it got rid of them and created the DV to encompass both. *Remember the DV.* The DV is what is placed on all foods and beverages—as well as vitamins/minerals/supplements that list nutrients on the label. It is supposed to represent the optimum amounts of nutrients applicable to the vast majority of Americans and is based on a 2,000 calorie/day diet.

In summary, the *only* acronym you need to remember is the DV. The previous four are no longer in existence except, maybe, in now outdated articles and textbooks. The changes were primarily due to a demand by a more health-conscious public for more specific guidelines.

* * *

One nongovernmental entity you need to know is the Food and Nutrition Board of the National Research Council of the Institute of Medicine of the National Academy of Sciences. Call it FNB for short. This is a private agency composed of scientists who set nutritional standards in the United States. The FNB also has five acronyms that relate to nutrient intake.

DRI

*D*ietary *R*eference *I*ntakes. This is a collective term that means nothing by itself. The term includes all of the following four acronyms. As I present the acronyms, they will be stated in *ascending* quantity of nutrients.

AI

*A*dequate *I*ntake. This is the clinically observed or experimentally derived intake for a specific population group that appears to maintain health. "Specific groups" would include each gender, various age groups within each gender, and various activity levels of age groups within each gender. It is *not* the absolute minimum to avoid maladies. It is more than that.

EAR

*E*stimated *A*verage *R*equirement. It is the estimated nutrient need of 50 percent of the individuals within a specific group. For example, if you took a specific group of say, sedentary females between the ages of twenty-one and forty, the EAR would be the nutrient amount that 50 percent of that group would exceed and 50 percent of that group would not exceed.

RDA

*R*ecommended *D*ietary *A*llowance. This is the nutrient amount that is perfectly adequate for 97 to 98 percent of all healthy adults in America. In other words, the vast majority of us do *not* need nutrients in excess of the RDA. Note that RDA is not the same as *USRDA* (above). The nutrient amounts are different; the "D" in RDA stands for "Dietary" as opposed to "Daily" in the USRDA; and, of course, RDA and USRDA are derived from different agencies—the RDA is private while the USRDA is a government group.

UL

Tolerable *U*pper Intake *L*evel. This is the "*Do not exceed*" level. If you do, there is at least a fifty-fifty chance you will suffer some toxic effects.

*　　*　　*

In summary, you may need to remember all of the FNB's acronyms, but be advised that the actual amounts of all nutrients may not be entirely available at the present time. Some already are available.

Don't despair. What I have done for you is to create a nifty chart that will show you the suggested lower limits; optimum amounts; and safe, upper limits.

If you've really been paying attention in this chapter, you may have suddenly got a bad case of whiplash if you snapped your head up and said, "*Wait a minute!* What good are all the books, acronyms, charts, and everything else if the absorption rates are not included? Doc, you told us that every vitamin has a different absorption rate and no vitamin is 100 percent absorbed. Are you telling me that I have to go find the absorption rates for every vitamin and then compute that relative to all the nutrient amounts that are given?"

Ahhhhhh, terrific questions. *In point of fact, the DVs, the RDAs, and everything on my charts do include the absorption rates.* You need to make no "allowance" for absorption rates. I've already done that for you.

In the amounts I list below, you should know that they do not necessarily equal amounts for DV, RDA, UL, or any other acronym (as I also said, some of the amounts are not out yet). What I did was to take all the research I could find, and erring on the side of (nonpolitical) conservatism, I have listed all amounts with built-in "safety factors." This was done so that you should feel comforted that if you stay within the "Minimum Requirements" and "Upper Limits," you should not suffer from any vitamin deficiency—from too little—or vitamin toxicity—from too much. You never need to exceed the "Optimum Amount" unless your physician says you need to do so. Don't self-prescribe. Remember, going below the minimum requirement—even for a few weeks with no replacement—will not make you keel over.

Look at the chart below and note the words used in the second, third, and fourth column headings. "Minimum Requirement" is the amount you should not go below. If you do, over a period of weeks or months, there appears to be a fifty-fifty chance you will suffer some malady due to that vitamin deficiency. "Optimum Amount" is the amount you should never need to exceed unless your physician tells you to do so. Individuals who might need to exceed the

"Optimum Amount" might be those recovering from major trauma, burns, an operation, or a fracture as well as certain conditions that are limited to the ladies (but only for specific situations) or true, strict vegetarians. If you have any doubts, talk to your physician!

Vitamin	Minimum Requirement	Optimum Amount	Upper Limit
Retinol A	800 IU	1,000 IU	5,000 IU
Beta Carotene	5,000 IU	25,000 IU	15,000 IU
B_1 Thiamine	.8 mg	2.0 mg	6.7 mg
B_2 Riboflavin	.8 mg	1.7 mg	6.9 mg
Niacin	5 mg	20 mg	35 mg
B_6 Pyridoxine	0.5 mg	2 mg	50 mg
Biotin	30 mcg	100 mcg	2,000 mcg
Pantothenic Acid	3.1 mg	10 mg	100 mg
Folic Acid	150 mcg	400 mcg	1,000 mcg
B_{12} Cobalamin	2 mcg	6 mcg	37 mcg
C	20 mg	60 mg	2,000 mg
D	80 IU/2 mcg	400 IU/10 mcg	2,000 IU/50 mcg
E Tocopherol	15 IU/2 mg	30 IU/10 mg	200 IU/80 mg
K	15 mcg	80 mcg	250 mcg

Please note the amount columns for vitamins D and E. For reasons no one could explain, some research was done using IU (International Units) while others used mcg or mg (microgram and milligram). So, because you may wind up reading the same research I did, I include *both* units of measurement.

Okay, you know your body must have *at least* the Minimum Requirement if you don't have any of the maladies associated with too little intake, or more than the Upper Limit if you don't have the toxicity associated with excessive intake. The question then becomes "How much do I really have?"

Here's how to find out. Take some sheets of paper or a small notebook. For each of the next thirty days simply jot down what you eat and drink for each day. At the end of thirty days, get a book and figure out how much of each vitamin you consumed during that thirty-day period. When you get the totals for each vitamin, divide the figure by thirty to get a daily average.

Then *add* that figure to the Minimum Requirement from the chart above (since you know you have at least that much, assuming you are not ill). That will give you your closest approximation to the amounts you have in your body at any point in time, without the high-cost blood tests. The best book that lists all the vitamins in foods and drinks is the fourth edition of *Introduction to Nutrition, Exercise and Health*, edited by Drs. Frank I. Katch and William D. McArdle.

When you have gotten the total figures for each vitamin (Minimum Requirement plus average daily amount), enter that figure in the chart below. The chart is a listing of an acceptable range of values, with the range being 50 percent above and below the Optimum Amount from the chart above. If you fall within the range—unless your physician recommends otherwise—*you do not need any vitamin supplements.*

If your figure falls below the low end of the range but above the Minimum Requirement, see your physician. If it is above the upper end of the range, but below the Upper Limit, cut back your intake.

Vitamin	Minimum Requirement	Acceptable Range		Upper Limit
		Low	High	
Retinol A	800 IU	2,500 IU	7,500 IU	25,000 IU
Beta Carotene	1000 IU	2,500 IU	7,500 IU	15,000
B_1 Thiamine	.8 mg	1.0 mg	3.0 mg	6.7 mg
B_2 Riboflavin	.8 mg	.85 mg	2.55 mg	6.9 mg
Niacin	5 mg	10 mg	30 mg	35 mg
B_6 Pyridoxine	0.5 mg	1.0 mg	3.0 mg	50 mg
Biotin	30 mcg	50 mcg	150 mcg	2,000 mcg
Pantothenic Acid	3.1 mg	5 mg	15 mg	100 mg
Folic Acid	150 mcg	200 mcg	600 mcg	1,000 mcg
B_{12} Cobalamin	2 mcg	3 mcg	9 mcg	37 mcg
C	20 mg	30 mg	90 mg	2,000 mg
D	150 IU/2 mcg	200IU/5mcg (low) 600IU/15mcg (high)		2,000 IU/50 mcg
E Tocopherol	15 IU/2 mg	20 IU/5 mg (low) 60 IU/15 mg (high)		200 IU/80 mg
K	15 mcg	40 mcg	120 mcg	250 mcg

Here's another tip: Suppose you do need to take more of one or more vitamins but, when you go to the store, the only quantities are several times more than you need as a supplement. For example, suppose you only need to add 2.5 mg niacin, but they only come in 5 mg tablets. At/near the pharmacy section, you can buy pill cutters. They're very inexpensive little boxes with a blade on the inside. Just put the pill inside, close the cover, and the blade cuts the pill into any size you want.

WARNING: DO NOT APPLY THE AMOUNTS IN ANY OF THE CHARTS TO ANYONE UNDER AGE TWELVE.

They are not applicable to children under age twelve, just as many medications (for adults) are not applicable to children under twelve, because (a) no studies have been done on these children or (b) studies have been done and adult dosages adversely affect children under twelve.

Now I want to give you, for each vitamin, what each is necessary for and what maladies you can incur if you take below the Minimum Requirement ("too little") or above the Upper Limit ("too much"). The listings do not necessarily mean you will get all of the maladies, and keep in mind that these only apply to people over age twelve and any malady may be as much one of the existence of the malady as well as one of *degree* of the malady. Because everybody is different, the presence of the malady, in any degree, is serious. For other people, the presence is not serious until the malady reaches a certain level. It varies by each person.

Vitamin A

Necessary for: Resistance to infections, formation of rhodopsin (the visual purple—a pigment in the outer segment of the retinal rods), prevention of night blindness, maintaining the epithelial tissues (the outer surfaces of the body and the linings of the surfaces of tubes leading to the exterior of the body, specifically sweat glands, oil glands, and salivary glands).

Too little: Retarded growth, susceptibility to infection, skin dryness, night blindness, xeropthalmia (severe dryness of the mucous membranes of the eyeball).

Too much: Nausea, vomiting, diarrhea, abdominal pain, hair loss, drying/cracking skin, itching and cracking of the lips, brittle finger- and toenails, loss of hemoglobin and potassium from red blood cells, cessation of menstruation, drowsiness, visual impairment, partial or total loss of appetite, muscle weakness, headaches, overall fatigue, enlargement of the liver and spleen, liver damage (including jaundice), marked increases in blood levels of triglycerides.

Vitamin B$_1$ (Thiamine)

Necessary for: Assistance in carbohydrate metabolism, maintenance of normal digestion and appetite, and the normal functioning of the tissues that carry nerve impulses.

Too little: Loss of appetite, digestion of starches and sugars is impaired, nervous disorders, beriberi, paralysis in men, loss of muscle coordination, colitis, constipation, diarrhea, and emaciation.

Too much: There are no known consistently recurring toxicity responses.

Vitamin B$_2$ (Riboflavin)

Necessary for: Normal growth, adaptation to light, formation of certain enzymes and oxidation of the cells, preventing cheilosis (a morbid reddening of the lips with the skin fissures at angles) and glossitis (inflammation of the tongue).

Too little: Impaired growth, glossitis, cheilosis, atrophy of the skin, cataracts, anemia, overall weakness, and photophobia (an unusual intolerance of light).

Too much: There are no known consistently recurring toxicity responses.

Niacin

Necessary for: Glycolysis, tissue respiration, fat synthesis, prevention of pellagra, and assists in vasodilation of blood vessels.

Too little: Dry, scaly, and crusty skin; development of cysts and ulcers; neurological and mental symptoms.

Too much: Abdominal cramps, nausea, vomiting, diarrhea, headaches, itching, decreased normal liver function, production of higher than normal levels of blood sugar.

B$_6$ (Pyridoxine)

Necessary for: Tryptophan (an essential amino acid necessary for normal growth and development) metabolism and utilization of some other amino acids.

Too little: Anorexia, dermatitis around the eyes and mouth, nausea and vomiting, and neuritis.

Too much: Irreversible nerve damage, especially the sensory nerves.

Biotin

Necessary for: Formation of fatty acids and energy-releasing reactions (energy metabolism).

Too little: Deficiency is extraordinarily rare—with extremely bizarre eating habits (primarily gorging oneself on raw egg whites!), but would result in depression, sleepiness, nausea, loss of appetite, and muscle pain, scaly skin, hair loss, swollen and dark-red tongue.

Too much: Almost no evidence that an excess is harmful.

Pantothenic Acid

Necessary for: Synthesis of sterols and steroid hormones and the central emphasis of energy metabolism.

Too little: Almost no evidence that any deficiency maladies exist.

Too much: Almost no evidence that an excess is harmful.

Folic Acid

Necessary for: The normal functioning of the hematopoietic system (which develops the red blood cells).

Too little: Anemia.

Too much: Nervous irritation, insomnia, and gastrointestinal distress.

B$_{12}$ (Cobalamin)

Necessary for: Conversion of folate into the form it can be used for production of red blood cells and nucleic acids for DNA synthesis.

Too little: Pernicious anemia, especially in true vegetarians.

Too much: No known effect of taking too much.

Vitamin C

Necessary for: Healing of wounds and fractures of bones, facilitates absorption of iron, prevention of scurvy, formation of intracellular cement substances in most tissues.

Too little: Lowered infection resistance, anemia, scurvy, hemorrhage, tenderness of the joints, bleeding gums and other dental problems (especially in oral tissues).

Too much: Diarrhea, nausea, abdominal cramps, headaches, fatigue, hot flashes, catalyst of gout, hemolytic anemia.

Vitamin D

Necessary for: The regulation of the absorption of calcium and phosphorous from the intestinal tract, and serves as an antirachitic (prevention of rickets).

Too little: Irritability, rickets, increased incidence of softening of bones and bone fractures, and tooth decay.

Too much: Disturbed calcium metabolism (leading to hypertension, nausea, loss of appetite), extensive kidney damage (leading to reabsorption of calcium causing formation of calcium crystals in the kidneys, which results in general weakness, vomiting, diarrhea, and greatly increased urine flow).

Vitamin E (Tocopheral)

Necessary for: Antioxidization in the fat-soluble portion of the cells, maintaining the integrity of the lungs and red blood cells.

Too little: Red blood cell resistance to rupture is decreased, and anemia.

Too much: Muscle weakness, overall fatigue, nausea, diarrhea, and abdominal pain.

Vitamin K

Necessary for: The synthesis of proteins necessary for blood coagulation.

Too little: Prolonging of blood-clotting time.

Too much: Muscle weakness, overall fatigue, nausea, diarrhea, and abdominal pain.

Read the following s-l-o-w-l-y. It is a summary of the *possible* benefits from some of the various vitamins. Understand that the evidence is *inconclusive* and also shows *only* that the vitamins *may*—not will—provide the benefits and has only proven that inconclusively in very small studies. Additional research is needed in all areas, so do not take what is stated as universal fact. It is not.

Vitamin A: May be of assistance in the fight against certain cancers and heart disease.

Niacin: Potential use as one preventive measure against diabetes.

Vitamin B$_6$: In conjunction with folic acid and vitamin B$_{12}$, it may help lower high levels of blood homocysteine (an amino acid), which has been associated with an increased risk of heart disease. Reduce symptoms of PMS.

Folic Acid: May reduce the risk of heart disease, colon and rectal cancers, the growth of precancerous cells of the cervix, depression, and deficiencies in learning and memory.

Vitamin B$_{12}$: Same as for vitamin B$_6$ (as to working in conjunction with other nutrients).

Vitamin C: May reduce the risk of heart disease, some cancers, and cataracts. May slightly lessen the duration of a cold, as well as some of the symptoms.

Vitamin D: May be used in the treatment of some disorders such as cancer.

Vitamin E: May improve the immune system and help fight heart disease, some cancers, Alzheimer's disease, and cataracts.

It is this area of possible benefits of vitamins, more than any other, where the hucksters misuse the evidence. They take this inconclusive evidence and do one or two things (or both) with the evidence. First, they will take one small, inconclusive factoid and create a sound bite that generalizes to the whole population. An example is, "Take vitamin E. Fight cancer." Or, they will make you feel insecure by saying, "Do you want to take a chance with your own life?" Most of us are so afraid of cancer that we'll rush out to buy vitamin E. The sales figures prove that's exactly what we have done.

They do this without telling you what amount would constitute an insufficient amount not to derive the benefits or the correct amount to derive the benefits. Second, they structure the ad to make you believe (a) your body does not have a sufficient level of the vitamin; (b) you won't get the benefits of the vitamin unless you take sufficient quantities of the vitamin; and (c) only their product is so "all-natural, scientifically advanced, balanced-formula, maximum-absorption, time-release capsulization . . ." that you will never be able to realize your life's potential of financial, religious, and sexual fulfillment unless you buy their product.

You may chuckle at what I have just said, but look at the ads and tell me how far off the mark you think I am (if at all).

*   *   *

The hucksters go from the sublime to the ridiculous when they tell us that we can even rub the vitamins into our body. Take some of the ads that say that the manufacturer's hair shampoo contains certain vitamins (usually, at least, vitamin E). It *is* true that hormones and nutrition are the most important factors—after genetics—that affect hair growth and density. The nutrition comes from *within* the body and is carried through the bloodstream to the hair bulb and follicle, which are below the outer layer of the scalp. The hucksters want you to believe—and we do believe it through the power of implication (without knowledge)—that somehow the vitamins are absorbed by the hair shaft (and maybe work their way down the shaft to the bulb and follicle) and make the hair more dense and shinier. Not true. This has never—I repeat, never—been proven. In fact, the "transport system" within the hair shaft—the medulla, cortex, cuticle cells, epithelial root sheath, etc.—are all designed to send cellular and sub-cellular matter *up and out* the shaft, not down and into it.

I earlier alluded to special groups that might have a legitimate need for additional nutrients above the DV, RDA, or my Optimum Amount. You may well fit into one of these groups if you are: pregnant; lactating; recovering from major surgery, a bone fracture, or burns; post-menopausal and over age sixty-five; a pure vegetarian; and, for whatever reason, know that you are not getting even the minimum amounts of vit-amins required. If you think about it, except for the pure vegetarian, you should either be under the care of a licensed physician or you need to be. Thus, you need to let your personal physician determine your cur-rent health status, and then let her/him tell you what, if any, vitamins you need to increase, by what amount, and for what length of time. Don't let some person who doesn't even know you exist try to shove them down your throat, however attractive the message, the packaging, the financial "deals" or "incentives," or the people in the ads.

I can't show the ads—at least by name of the manufacturers—but I can present the wording that appears at the bottom of some of them, especially those on the Internet. I can't show the full ad *because* of the wording, which appears at the very bottom of the ads, which says the ad is copyrighted and may not be reproduced. I present a synopsis of the wording in many of those ads. I have itali-cized certain words for emphasis:

Legal Terms and Conditions

We restrict the use of the contents of this advertisement, make *no* warranties or representations about the *accuracy or completeness* at, in or connected to this site, and *nobody* can hold us liable for *any* damages for *any* reason.

Oh, that's great. That's outstanding. Someone makes all kinds of claims about a nutritional product then totally disavows *everything*. If you're thinking I'm making up all of this, get on the Internet, type in "vitamins" on a search engine, pull up the ad, scroll to the bottom, and see for yourself.

And you still want to spend your money on products like that? Please don't.

Take a look at the ads that follow. See if you can notice where the ads go astray of the whole truth. I think you'll be surprised at how good you'll be at it.

The first ad is for a company called Natural-Vitamin.com.[2] Look at the wording just to the right of *Natural Vitamins*. "The power of nature" is an incredibly broad statement. It's so broad as to be meaningless, except to condition you for what follows. "Improve your life!" is nice, but it doesn't say in what areas, or by what amounts, or how to measure it. "Feel better with quality all-natural products. . . ." Feel better than what? When? For how long? Remember, I said "all-natural" is an industry-created phrase. It has no accepted definition in medicine or science. "Natural" means the way it occurs or exists in nature. This means vitamins that exist in their natural state, as in an orange, a piece of meat, a head of lettuce, etc. Even if the ad said "natural" instead of "all-natural" it would mean as I state it in the previous sentence, but by some strange transfer of logic, they refer to "all-natural" as nutrients in pills and tablets. This is peculiar, and it's not true. I repeat, a vitamin is a vitamin is a vitamin or it is not. It is simply a consistent chemical chain that makes a particular vitamin, and if that chemical chain (or bond) changes, the vitamin is no longer the vitamin it was. Natural or synthetic, they're all the same!

Then the ad continues in the next section with "Uncover your bodies [*sic*] full potential. . . ." This is truly a piece of work. First, where has your potential been hiding so that you can only uncover it with the products listed on this Web site? Second, the word "bodies" (which is a plural usage—maybe it works for mutants) should be the possessive case, "body's." How do you measure when you have your "full potential"? And is this a singular measurement, or multiple as in mental, psychological, physical . . . what? The same applies to the meaningless general phrase "improve performance." The ad is a classic example of unfounded statements, generalizations, and incomplete implications that, when you complete them, you wind up duping yourself.

I love the next ad, for a KareMor Product Line.[3] They offer spray vitamins and nutritional supplements. Please look at the ad. First of all, their opening salvo heralds "A truetechnological [their word(s)] breakthrough that's revolutionizing. . . ." Recall that I cautioned you at the beginning of this discussion to ignore any ads with that type of wording. Second, try as I might, I can find no evidence on just what the "Nutritional Advisory Council" is, or who sits on that council.

Third, the ad says, ". . . millions of Americans are taking vitamin pills that may be doing them little, if any, good." I agree! But I agree because we don't need them. Their point isn't made until the next paragraph when the wheels really come off their wagon. I know of *no evidence* that any vitamin pill goes through your digestive system

---

Natural-Vitamin.com

Vitamins

Sports & Weight Loss

Herbs & Herbal Teas

If you are searching for any of the following topics:

- vitamins
- vitamin supplements
- buy vitamins online
- vitaminn online

Nutritional Food Supplements

Look no further. You'll find it at Natural-Vitamin.com!

Natural Vitamins

Use the power of nature to improve your life! Feel better with quality all-natural products from Natural-Vitamin.com

Personal Care

Only quality products make it on our site. Uncover your bodies full potenial and improve performance. Buy online from the comfort and privacy of your home! Huge selection to choose from.

At Natural-Vitamin.com, you'll discover an easy to use, information packed web site. Click here to learn more.

Get the Know How here

Shop-Online

Shop Online

Let's Spray Health
KareMor Product Line

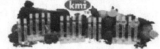

KareMor Independent Distributor
Tel (813) 989-0167 - Fax (813) 987-2541

Spray Vitamins & Nutritional Supplements: A truetechnological breakthrough that's revolutionizing the vitamin and nutritional supplement industry!

Content & Purity 100 % Certified By The Nutritional Advisory Council

Today in America, more than 169 million people take vitamins or some type of nutritional supplement.

The startling fact is that millions of Americans are taking vitamin pills that may be doing them little, if any, good.

Why? Because many vitamin pills do not dissolve in the digestive tract quickly enough to be absorbed. In addition, by the time the digestive process is completed, it has been proven that *only a small percentage* of the nutrient actually enters the bloodstream!

Spray nutrients solve the problem!

This chart is from the most recent edition of the prestigious Physician's Desk Reference manual tells the story!

so fast that it isn't absorbed. But they make that statement and then contradict themselves by saying, ". . . *only a small percentage* of the nutrient actually enters the bloodstream!" Hold it right there! Look, if the pill *never* dissolved in your digestive system, *none* of it would get in your bloodstream. But the ad says, ". . . it has been proven. . . ." Baloney. If there is nothing that occurs in the digestive system, the percentage is *real* small. It's spelled z-e-r-o.

Now the ad states that you can spray the nutrients into your mouth to get a real quick absorption. Why do you want to do that? Your body already has the nutrients in it (or you'd probably be in a hospital if the amount were truly zero). Getting the nutrients "dispensed throughout your body in seconds" is not important. Your health or life does not depend on that speed of nutrient absorption. Whoever wrote the ad needs some coursework in anatomy and phys-

From The Physician's Desk Reference

Oral Absorption Rate is Nine Times Better Than Pills!

100% It clearly illustrates the superior results provided by oral sprays.

How does oral absorption work? Pure nutritional molecules are absorbed into the body through the lining of the mouth. Blood capillaries are extremely close to the surface in this area. This highly absorbent tissue allows nutrients to be absorbed into the bloodstream where they are dispensed throughout the body in seconds.

AMOUNT ABSORBED

PILL · GEL-CAPSULE · TRANSDERMAL PATCH · SUBLINGUAL LIQUID · INTRAMUSCULAR INJECTION · INTRA-ORAL SPRAY

METHOD OF DELIVERY

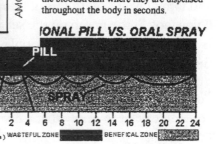

IONAL PILL VS. ORAL SPRAY

PILL

SPRAY

0 2 4 6 8 10 12 14 16 18 20 22 24
Time (Hours) WASTEFUL ZONE ▮▮ BENEFICAL ZONE ▨▨

NO MORE PEAKS AND VALLEYS

peaks and valleys? When a pill first dissolves, too much nutrient is released into the system creating a "peak". In fact, if the tablet dissolves, (and many do not!) nutrients may be washed out of the system as waste. As time goes on, too little nutrients are available and the body experiences a "valley". This chart from a prestigious Pharmacological Journal illustrates how sprays eliminate the "peaks and valleys".

LET'S TRY OUR CURRENT PRODUCT LINE

Click Here For KareMor Order Center

- Vitamist Performance (More Info.)
- Advance Performance (More Info.)
- Extend Performance (More Info.)
- Renew Performance (More Info.)

- VitaSight (NEW) (More Info.)
- VitaZac (NEW) (More Info.)
- DHEA-W (for women only) (NEW) (More Info.)
- DHEA-M (for men only) (NEW) (More Info.)
- VitaMinophen (Pain Reliever) (More Info.)
- Ladymate (NEW) (More Info.)
- Vitamist Adult Multiple (More Info.)
- CardioCare (NEW) (More Info.)
- Vitamist Children's Multiple (More Info.)
- Vitamist Prenatal (More Info.)
- Vitamist B-12 (More Info.)
- Vitamist C+Zinc (More Info.)

iology. Here's why. Even when the nutrients are sprayed into your mouth and begin tooling around in your blood vessels, you will feel nothing—no burst of energy, no flash of mental brilliance, no sudden disease cure. Nothing. However, because the nutrients are in your bloodstream, they go where blood goes. And your blood flows through your digestive system, where the liver and kidneys do yeoman work. And if the body doesn't need the nutrients as it goes through these "processing plants" it either stores them or excretes them. No other options are possible. The ad's selling points about the implied urgent need for quick absorption and small percentage actually entering the bloodstream are meaningless.

Have you ever looked in the *Physician's Desk Reference*? It's a big book. Thousands of drugs are cross-referenced, given by generic and formal name, with lots of information about each one. However, if you look at the graph on the second page of the ad, the implication is that the graph is referring only to nutrients. That is false. In fact, the reference is primarily to over-the-counter and prescription drugs. Vitamins and minerals are *not* drugs. Also, just compare absorption rates of transdermal patches to intra-oral sprays. Be careful. I'm sure you don't want to imply that a nicotine spray is more effective than a transdermal patch. Truthfully, substances such as nicotine and cyanide occur *naturally* in nature—and they can both kill you (and I don't mean over a long period of time. I'm talking mere minutes, if you absorbed them in a condensed, pure form). In fact, some drugs are forbidden to be administered by a spray, regardless of where on your body it is applied.

Now take a look at the ad for "Comprehensive Formula."[4] They lose it in the first paragraph. Energy does not come from the nutrients listed on the page. Energy comes from calories, as found in fat, carbohydrate, and protein. *Vitamins and minerals contain no energy*. In energy metabolism, they are released by the protein, carbohydrate, and fat, in that order as the length of exercise/movement goes from seconds to minutes. There is overlap as time progresses, meaning that, while fats really begin to be utilized as the source of energy after approximately twenty minutes of exercise/movement, it does *not* mean that no fat is used at the 19:59 mark and only fat is utilized at the 20:00 mark.

Then they do a header with the ". . . finest quality ingredients. . . ." As you now know, all vitamins are the same and the rest is filler. And filler is inert. Quality is irrelevant because there can be no difference or the nutrient is something else. And, when they get down to "Natural vitamin E," there is no way of determining if it's "More potent, easier to absorb, and better tolerated . . ." than any-

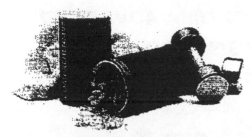

Comprehensive Formula

Comprehensive Formula will give you the essential nutrients known to improve your health and give you energy!

With Comprehensive Formula you get thirty vitamins and minerals in one. It's simple, complete and balanced with the finest quality ingredients.

Antioxidants Combat Free-Radical Damage

Comprehensive Formula provides the highest quality and optimum amounts of all major antioxidant nutrients:

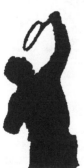

- **Natural vitamin E**
  More potent, easier to absorb, and better tolerated than the much cheaper synthetic form commonly found in vitamin supplements. And a full 200 IU, many times more than Centrum or One-A-Day.

- **Vitamin A with mixed natural carotenoids**
  A rich mixture of natural beta-carotene which has been shown to be a greater antioxidant than the common synthetic type, plus the full spectrum of natural carotenoids, many of which appear to be more powerful antioxidants than beta-carotene. Also includes 50% of the Daily Value (DV) of vitamin A Palmitate - a safe and effective level to supplement your diet. Plus, 500 mg. of vitamin C - considered the most important antioxidant vitamin for humans. Vitamin C has been shown to provide valuable health benefits at levels well above the RDA of 60 mg. and selenium - two different forms for maximum absorption, retention, and utilization.

- **B vitamin maintain physical and mental well-being**
  B vitamins are essential for peak physical and mental performance. They metabolize food into energy and maintain the health of your cardiovascular and nervous systems. Because the typical American diet is deficient in many B vitamins, Comprehensive Formula provides amounts greater than the minimum RDAs. The men's formula contains higher levels of vitamins B2, niacin, B12 and pantothenic acid, due to men's greater needs.

About Comprehensive | Ingredients | Specially Formulated | Our Offer

SYNERGY OPTIMA ADVANCED
Ingredients
DARE TO COMPARE !!!!!

LOOK AT OUR DOUBLE GUARANTEE!!!! GUARANTEED LOWEST PRICE! GUARANTEED MAXIMUM NUTRITION IN ONE BOTTLE!	9 Caplets Daily: Taken 3 Caplets, 3 times per day, prior to or with meals supply	% of US RDA	Use this column to compare any other brand
Vitamins			
Ascorbyl Palmitate (Lipid Soluble Vitamin C)	100 mg	70	
Beta Carotene	25,000 IU	500	
Biotin	150 mcg	50	
Folic Acid	400 mg	100	
Niacin	25 mg	125	
Niacinamide	100 mg	500	
Pantothenic Acid (d-Calcium Pantothenate)	50 mg	500	
Vitamin A (Acetate)	5000 IU	100	
Vitamin B-1 (Thiamine HCL)	50 mg	3333	
Vitamin B-2 (Riboflavin)	20 mg	1176	
Vitamin B-6 (Pyrodoxine HCL)	20 mg	1000	
Vitamin B-12 (Cobalamin Concentrate)	30 mcg	500	
Vitamin C (Ascorbic Acid)	1500 mg	2500	
Vitamin D-3 (Cholecalciferol)	200 IU	50	
Vitamin K (Phytonadione)	70 mcg	**	
Vitamin E Complex			
Vitamin E (d-Alpha-Tocopherol Acetate)	300 IU	1000	

thing else, because there is no comparison to anything, except this mysterious "... cheaper synthetic form ..." and we never know what that is.

They then proceed through the same, tired litany of claims about health benefits, peak performance, etc. Pardon me while I yawn at their futile efforts.

Near the bottom of the page, they make the unproven statement that ". . . the typical American diet is deficient in many B vitamins. . . ." Nice try with creating a panic, but it's not true. At the bottom of the page, the ad says, "The men's formula contains higher levels of vitamins B2, niacin, B12 and pantothenic acid, due to men's greater needs."True. What they don't tell you is that—except for iron—every single vitamin and mineral requirement is equal to, or greater, for men than women and that is true across all age groups. If you simply follow my charts, the DV, or the RDA, they *already* take into account those differences (as well as the absorption rates, as previously mentioned).

And we come, some might say mercifully, to the last ad for this chapter, one for "Synergy Optima Advanced."[5] They're trying to put as many whiz-bang words in the title as possible. Big deal. They dare us to compare. Okay, let's take them up on the dare. Just do it for the vitamins.

Here's how you do it. Go to my charts and take the figures in the Minimum Requirement column. Add to this the amount that you computed as your daily average intake over a thirty-day period (if you haven't done it yet, please do so, but go ahead and keep reading and come back and do the comparison after you compute your thirty-day averages). Then add the amounts the ad lists in its second column. When you get the totals of those three figures, go back to my second chart and look at the Acceptable Range (High and Low) column. If the total of the three figures exceeds the "High" figure in the Acceptable Range, you're really wasting it, and you may well find some figures exceed the Upper Limit! In fact, some of their amounts—by themselves, *without* any addition for what's already in your body plus what you ingest on a daily basis—*exceed* the Upper Limits. That is dangerous territory. It makes no sense to put yourself at risk, when all you have to do is verify that you are within a pretty wide range of amounts.

The ad actually had more pages, but I limited the presentation just to what is relevant to vitamins.

VIPS

All vitamins are simply chemicals, whether produced by nature or in a laboratory.

Vitamins contain no energy; the body regulates the amount of energy released; and no increase in consumption of vitamins will result in a corresponding increase in the energy in, or produced by, the body.

According to the American Dietetic Association, smoking, stress, or exercise do not "rob" the body of any vitamins.

All vitamins are absorbed at less than 100 percent, with the highest level of absorption occurring when vitamins are in their natural position in foods and liquids, and these absorption rates always exceed absorption rates of synthetic vitamins.

The average retail price markup of vitamins exceeds 400 percent; 1300 percent for a single RDA dose; and the whole-sale cost of the RDA of all the vitamins in one capsule is less than one cent.

The contents of all vitamin pills or tablets produced synthetically are mostly filler.

You only need to know the vitamin amounts contained in DV, RDA, or, most simply, my charts.

The next chapter is especially important because there are some real problems with mineral deficiencies in humans. In point of fact, most of the problems affect women.

And too much of certain minerals can—and have—killed people.

NOTES

1. F. I. Katch and W. D. McArdle, *Introduction to Nutrition, Exercise and Health*, 4th ed. (Baltimore, Md.: Williams & Wilkins, 1993).

2. Natural-Vitamin.com. Internet advertisement printed from address http://www.natural-vitamin.com/nutrition/ [14 August 1999], p. 1.

3. KareMor Product Line. Internet advertisement printed from address

http://zipmall.com/letspray/karemor/products.htm [14 August 1999], pp. 1–2 of 3.

4. Comprehensive Formula. Internet advertisement printed from address http://www.buyitontheweb.com/cgibin/buyit/comprehensive/index? L6nxPqXx;;3 [19 July 1999], p. 1 of 1.

5. Optima Advanced. Internet advertisement printed from address http://www.nutrimax.pair.com/ingredients.htm [19 July 1999], p. 1 of 3.

5

MINERALS
Women *Are* at Risk Here

My confidential ad industry source also told me that the industry made plans for a big emphasis on minerals starting in 2000. He said that ad executives were becoming fearful that vitamins were getting overexposed to, and better understood by, the general public. Those executives thought the easy money had been made on vitamins and it was time to shift to a more financially fertile focus. He added that people are much less knowledgeable about minerals and are, therefore, much more susceptible and gullible to ads about minerals. He concluded by stating that the formats of ads are changing—as always with the most subtle of assaults.

When you tune in a station, turn on a channel, or open a magazine, you transport yourself—untutored—into an alien culture; one based on deceit. Greed is the knife that separates truth from fiction. If those two sentences were not obvious to you before you started to read this book, they should now be thunderingly clear. Taken a step further, when feeling—not fact—becomes the basis for the advertising culture, truth is shattered and is unlikely to be recovered. Statements such as "I feel better," "I feel more alert," "I feel younger," "I feel I need more nutrients," "I feel stronger"—all without proof (especially quantitative proof)—are the siren songs of seduction that separate you from your money. The hucksters will argue that they need more and more of these types of strategies and tactics to survive in the "competitive marketplace," when all they are doing is employing twisted logic to get themselves off the hook for their own actions.

The demand for your attention has gotten so frantic, you are now (or soon will be) assaulted by even more insipid audio and visual "grabbers."

The latest tactics are as follows: If you are watching TV or are on the Internet you will get hit with "blinkers." Blinkers are words or pictures that flash continually during the ad, designed to continually "grab" the focus of your eyes and move them to a specific part of the ad. This occurs even though the vocal portion may be talking about something else, but the spoken words can be a reinforcement of that which is blinking and not in competition with it.

Additionally, TV ads hit you with "flashers." Flashers occur when there is a switch from one camera to another. As the switch occurs, a flash, exactly like that of a flashbulb, assaults your eyes. Again, this is meant to jerk your eyes back to the ad. Can you imagine how long you would continue to read this book if, on every page, a portion of it was a continual blinking sentence and, every time you turned the page, a flashbulb went off in your face?

People are actually getting nauseous from these ads. Here's why: The camera switching/flashing usually occurs at the rate of one to three times per second. When people are subjected to flashing/blinking lights at a specific rate (called a "frequency"), they suffer what is called "flicker vertigo." It happens to pilots who fly propeller-driven aircraft, especially when the prop is on the nose of the aircraft and the plane is heading into the sun. As the prop turns, it passes in front of the sun, and you get a typical strobe light effect. Pilots have gotten flicker vertigo, become totally disoriented, lost control of the aircraft, and crashed. No one knows the range of frequencies that cause flicker vertigo. Oftentimes the ads overlay text and/or flashing with pounding rock music.

And, if pounding rock music weren't enough of an irritation while you're trying to listen to the words that are being spoken, the TV ad producers tie the flasher with another sound that reminds me of someone spitting up phlegm. If you've heard it (and Fox is notorious for doing this on sports programming), you may describe it as a guttural, tearing sound. As it applies to ads, this occurs when a scene shifts, there is a switch from one camera to another, or even when the ad just begins to run—the combination effect being to keep your eyes *and* ears from wandering off the focus of the ad. I laugh and cry at the situation as it relates to ads. I laugh because there is now a growing body of evidence that watching ads can literally make you sick. I cry because of the incredible callousness to which we suckers are being subjected, all in the name of money. Ads have gotten so disgusting in their attempts to force us to watch and listen, we wind up with a case of sensory overload.

So, while the lies and misrepresentations continue, now coupled with increasing infantile and frantic attempts to get and keep our attention, the product factually remains unchanged. What follows is the essential information regarding vitamins and minerals; exactly what hucksters *don't* want you to have.

There is a similarity and a difference between vitamins and minerals and these exist at the most basic level—that of the atoms. Both are chemical chains. Vitamins are organic substances, which means they always include carbon atoms. They exist in nature in animals, and in plants. Minerals are inorganic. They have no carbon atoms and also exist in nature but they do not exist naturally in animals or in plants. They are found in animals and plants *because* they consume the earth's water and/or topsoil that naturally contain the minerals. Minerals are usually in solid form and the best sources of minerals are animal products because minerals are more highly concentrated in animal tissues than in plants.

The cycle runs very much like this: Water, in the form of rain and melted snow, washes minerals into the soil where they then are carried beneath the soil. This mineral-laden water moves underground until, basically, one of two things happens: (1) roots of plants absorb that water, or (2) we "extract" the water from the ground (or it flows out freely) and drink it.

If we eat the plants, we consume minerals. If animals eat the plants and then we eat the animals, we consume minerals. If we drink the water, we consume minerals. When plants and animals die, their tissues decay, which causes the minerals to return to the soil to await the rain and the cycle begins anew.

* * *

Whereas vitamins exist to aid in activating chemical processes within the body (while *not* becoming a part of the reaction they help affect), minerals often become part of the structure and working chemicals of the body. For example, the mineral calcium becomes part of the bones. Additionally, minerals participate in the breakdown (catabolic) and buildup (anabolic) processes within the body's cells. They participate as regulators; i.e., they assist in the balance between the continual breaking down and building up of the cells and the resultant effects.

Remember in the previous chapter where I mentioned that the word "bioavailability" was used incorrectly regarding vitamins? It does refer to minerals; specifically, it refers to the amount of absorption of the mineral by the body. There's a more sensitive issue here. More so than vitamins, some minerals can *interact* with (complement) other minerals and some *compete* with other minerals. This is where the balance of "not too little, not too much" becomes critical. See if the information in the following paragraph confuses you. Better yet, see if you can even remember all of it (and be aware, I am presenting only a few of all the possible interactions).

For example, if your body consumes calcium in excess of its needs, it interferes with the absorption of iron and magnesium; too much zinc reduces the absorption of copper. Too much fiber decreases zinc absorption. A high-protein diet inhibits calcium absorption. Minerals also interact with vitamins to affect their absorption. For example, vitamin C increases the absorption of iron and vitamin D increases the absorption of calcium. Even drugs can cause changes in nutrient absorption. Oral contraceptives interfere with the metabolism of vitamins B_6, B_{12}, and folic acid—as does excessive consumption of alcohol. Got all that?

Here's the problem: If you start taking supplemental amounts of vitamins and minerals, you throw the body's natural—optimal and automatic—absorption rates out of whack. But the hucksters never tell you this. You could well be doing your body more harm than good by taking vitamins and minerals above amounts you need.

The previous statement, as much as anything, is the critical basis for what you keep hearing as a "balanced" diet. Perhaps this new perspective can be stated: *Let your body do what it was built to do naturally and stop throwing its natural balance out of whack by introducing additional substances in amounts it doesn't need and simply must work harder to process and eject.*

At this point, I am going to introduce the risks that women, especially, incur due to being women, and what to do about it. I think it will also aid in your attention when you read further as to specific minerals. *And, make no mistake about it, in the United States adult population, most nutrition deficiencies occur almost* exclusively *in women*.

Ladies, because you are women, you do things that men don't, and this puts you at higher risk. Here are some examples: You get pregnant, you breast-feed, you menstruate, you go through menopause, you diet to an extreme, you spend more time taking care of your children. The first four are physiological; the last two are not.

During a pregnancy, the fetus must obtain its nutrients from its mother. That draws down the nutrients normally available to the mother. Those nutrients are primarily zinc, iron, calcium, and folic acid.

The same fact holds true with breast-feeding.

When you menstruate, you lose blood. This causes a reduction of the total amount of iron stores in your body. The heavier the menstrual flow, the greater the loss of blood and, therefore, the loss of iron.

When you go through menopause, you are relieved of menstruation and its attendant loss of blood and iron, but the estrogen that was being produced in your body is greatly reduced; in some cases, production totally ceases. The result is that your bones begin to become porous, and you get osteoporosis (which literally means "porous bones"). This is because you are deficient in calcium. We're not exactly sure why the loss of estrogen has a concurrent loss of calcium, but it does happen.

In fact, anyone who suffers from any type of internal bleeding—and this includes people with ulcers—could well be deficient in iron.

When you go on extreme diets—which are defined as any diet where you take in fewer than 1,000 calories per day—the foods you ingest at that low-calorie level do not contain sufficient nutrients to supply your body with what it needs.

When you spend more time with your children—for better or worse—what happens to those children is mostly your responsibility. To illustrate my point, what would be your answer to this question: "What is the most common cause of infant poisoning deaths?" If you answered "insecticides," "alcohol," or "cleaning solvents," you would be wrong in each case. According the the American Dietetic Association, *the most common cause of infant poisoning deaths is the ingestion of iron supplements*. Hucksters will never tell you that.

Now, to specifics and quantitative amounts.

As to iron, you lose an average of 4 to 45 mg of your body's iron store during each menstrual cycle, depending on the menstrual flow. Since the average female ingests only 10.2 mg per day of iron, it's easy to suffer an iron deficit. In fact, 30 to 50 percent of all women exhibit significant iron deficiency, with a full 10 percent being truly anemic—not a good situation. Pregnancy results in an average of 10 to 15 mg per day being utilized by the fetus.

When you consider that the RDA for a young woman is 15 mg of iron per day, it's not difficult to see how quickly her complete daily intake could be totally depleted.

If your physician tells you to take iron supplements, take them with an eight-ounce glass of orange juice, because this will increase the absorption rate of the iron by 200 to 300 percent due to the folic acid in the juice. Only 2 to 20 percent of the iron from plants is absorbed by your body, while 10 to 35 percent is absorbed from animal meats (which include fish).

What is not well known is that approximately 10 percent of Americans are *genetically predisposed* to accumulate harmful amounts of iron. The caution here is that you should take iron supplements *only* under a physician's direction. *To do otherwise could kill you*. The hucksters never give you that warning.

Infant poisoning is due to parental carelessness. The FDA has no requirement for a warning label as to this fact in regards to iron supplements. Would it be too much to ask the manufacturers to place such a warning label on their iron supplement packaging about the genetic predisposition and infant safety?

Incidentally, if you are a female athlete, there is no conclusive evidence to prove that moderate-to-high levels of athletic training or exercise produce exercise-induced anemia (EIA), which has also been called "sports anemia."

More about calcium. To expand on what I mentioned above as to osteoporosis, when the body's intake of calcium is insufficient, it draws on calcium reserves within the body—in the bones—to replace the deficit. If this imbalance (deficit) is prolonged, osteoporosis occurs. When osteoporosis does occur, the bones get brittle and they break easily under the stress of normal living. This can be as mundane as sitting down, getting up from a chair, climbing steps, and getting in and out of a car.

Because the spine is made up of many bones, as those bones become porous, the spine actually shrinks to a noticeable degree, with the result that posture is severely affected (the unfortunate person is severely "hunched over") and the spine becomes unable to support the body in an upright posture.

Especially in women over the age of sixty, I would say that calcium deficiency has reached epidemic proportions. According to F. I. Katchard and W. D. McArdle, authors of *Introduction to Nutrition, Exercise and Health*, 4th ed., this is compounded by the fact that calcium absorption rarely exceeds 35 percent, and this absorption is inhibited by eating meat and salt, drinking alcohol and coffee (it doesn't matter whether it's decaffeinated or not), as well as smoking.

The latest statistics I have seen as to the (in)adequacy of calcium consumption are:

1. Approximately 25 percent of all females consume less than 300 mg on any given day, which is far less than the RDA of between 800 and 1,200 mg;
2. Approximately 75 percent of adults in the United States consume less than the RDA for calcium;
3. For females ages eleven to twenty-four, the recommended daily intake is 1,200 mg and 1,200 to 1,500 for postmenopausal women not on estrogen replacement therapy.

The hucksters in the health and fitness industry do not want to educate you. They might say so, but their actions speak otherwise. What they are doing is informing you. Informing is not education. Informing is merely presenting information. You don't know whether the information is factual or not. You aren't told how to prove or disprove the information. You aren't told whether the information applies directly to you or to the population in general.

I had some meetings with Mark Crossen in the spring of 1994. He was the CEO of a company called Amrion, which was a fledging manufacturer of supplements, located in Boulder, Colorado. I had entered into discussions with Crossen about his willingness to manufacture any specific combination of nutrients that I could test on patients to determine if they could make a person measurably younger. I had the testing mechanism available in my National Center for Sports Medicine in Denver, Colorado. My friend, Dr. John Sbabaro, was a full professor of Preventive Medicine at the University of Colorado Health Sciences Center as well as the director for the Center for Prevention. John graciously agreed to allow me the use of his facilities and some of his personnel at the Center for Prevention to conduct the study.

When I asked Crossen his company's philosophy, he told me that they came out with some new combination of nutrients every month to stay competitive and make it seem like new discoveries were being made monthly. I asked him if he felt it was his company's job to educate the consumer. He told me that it absolutely was not their job to educate the consumer. Their job was to make money for the company.

To truly educate someone, you must present them with independently verifiable facts—and it should be the *whole* story, not conveniently taken out of context—and not unsubstantiated opinion or political spin. I ask you at this point to stop for a moment and reflect if you believe you are getting fact (education) or information from the hucksters.

Incidentally, if you look on the front page of the Business Section of the *Rocky Mountain News*, on 28 May 1994, you will find a story about Crossen and Amrion. The FDA had nailed them for misleading labeling practices and Amrion had offered $500,000 to settle, which the FDA had refused. You know that something major was involved.

But all during the discussions with Dr. Sbabaro and me, Crossen had never let on that he was in trouble with the FDA. He just stopped returning our phone calls. Then we saw the story in the *Rocky Mountain News*. We never called him after that, for obvious reasons. I present this story as an example of what I have run into time and again on a professional basis.

Though you may not like our federal government, agencies such as the FDA generally do a very good job at their assigned task(s), even though this might be at cross-purposes with what politicians do. For example, former president Bill Clinton really caved in to the hucksters. In 1994 he signed into law the Dietary Supplement Health and Education Act. Notice the word "education" in the title; you'll see it was just the opposite from education that was signed into law. The act removed dietary supplements from premarket safety evaluations required of food ingredients and drugs. The act eliminated the FDA's authority to regulate the safety of nutritional supplements *before* they're on the market. Now, the FDA can only intervene *after* injury, illness, or death occurs, and only if the FDA can prove the harm occurred from taking the supplement "as directed."

Thus, the manufacturers can say *anything* they want before the supplement hits the market. The marketing reps (independent reps) can make any claim—even to saying something like, "It cures all types of cancer" or "Take this and you'll live thirty years longer, guaranteed" or "It will prevent every birth defect known to man"—as long as they're not selling the product at the same time. It doesn't take too much brainpower to deduce that the hucksters will lie through their teeth in a presentation, then sell you the product the next day. This way, they were not "selling you the product" at the *same* time the claims were made.

Once the product is on the market, the label on the product (which includes any packaging) cannot make any false or misleading claims. Unfortunately, the FDA readily admits it simply doesn't have the resources to pursue the thousands of complaints it gets each year, and this situation is getting markedly worse because of the explosion of false and misleading ads being generated over the Internet. As it stands now, you cannot be sure of either the purity or the amount of the ingredients from one package to the next, even for the *same* product from the *same* manufacturer! And, because of that, the price is no indicator of the quality or potency of the product. *The only way you can be relatively sure is if the product meets the voluntary standards of the U.S. Pharmacopeia* (a nonprofit body that sets quality standards for medicines for human and veterinary use) *for quality, purity, tablet dissolution, and tablet disintegration*. It will state this on the label.

Oftentimes you have no idea what the product is that you are purchasing or whether it is a "good" bargain. The following will illustrate my point.

☐ #10. THE PRINCIPLE OF IRRELEVANT OVERLOAD

The Principle of Irrelevant Overload is a practice of adding to, or including with, the ingredients of a product, where the additions may not only be unnecessary, they may even be harmful to you. This is not the same as adding a newsletter to a bottle of supplements "for the low, fantastic introductory one-time only offer. . . ."

Take a look at the following ad that was taken off the Internet on 12 September 1999. It's for a product called "Montmorillonite."[1] Big word. Do you have any idea what it means? I do. The named title of the product is also the name of the substance. Montmorillonite is a substance usually found underwater or under the earth's surface in long-dead plants. It is extremely mineral dense. That means it contains a lot of minerals.

Look at the ad. At "Description" those infamous words "all natural" are used. All natural, huh? Well, if you look at "Ingredients" it includes ". . . Raspberry or Chocolate flavoring and tableting aids." So much for "all natural" when you add artificial flavoring, and I have no idea what the "tableting aids" are. Do you?

The ad also states that "500 Mg of Montmorillonite with 67 Minerals. . . ." *67?*

Dear reader, the human body needs only 15 minerals, not 67. I'll be damned if I'm knowingly going to put anything in my body that contains 52 minerals that my body doesn't need, nor do I even know

Montmorillonite

Montmorillonite: (Chewable) An Important source of Calcium, Selenium, Vanadium, Chromium, Manganese, Magnesium, and Zinc.

Description: Montmorillonite trace minerals are an all natural combination of colloidal silicate minerals which are nature's storehouse for the largest group of chemical elements in the mineral kingdom. Motmorillonite contains over 188 mineral compounds in micro-amounts and over 66 minerals.

As a dietary supplement, users report improvement of health in many areas such as more energy and stamina, reduced arthritis pain, stronger and faster growing nails, thicker hair, stronger teeth, fewer cavities, healing of bleeding gums, faster healing of wounds or fractures, fewer colds, smoother complexion, better weight control, and an overall healthier body.

Ingredients: 500 Mg of Montmorillonite with 67 Minerals and trace elements, fructose, Raspberry or Chocolate flavoring and tableting aids.

120 ct. Chewable Tablets (chocolate or raspberry)
500 mg.

Retail Price: $32.50   **Distributor's Price: $27.50** (monthly autoship)

Click Here To Order This Or Any Other Product

Othoer Herbs:

Vital-Food
Vital-Burn
Vital-Energy
Vital-Mind
Vital-Antioxidant
NuZac (Nature's Answer To Prozac)

---

what those extra 52 minerals are. You see, the hucksters are informing (not educating) and they are offering you this "mineral rich" substance. They don't tell you that you don't need 52 of them, so there is your "irrelevant overload." *Don't assume more is better.* It is also not stated how much of any of the 67 minerals are included per tablet. Amazing.

The ad does use a word you may also not be familiar with—"colloidal." Think that sounds high-tech? Maybe on the frontiers of new scientific knowledge? Something that makes the product just too good to pass up? Think again. The root word is "colloid." It means something that is a uniform mixture in a structure. In this context it is a way of describing montmorillonite, because a supplement made from colloids contains in excess of sixty minerals. Look familiar?

Hucksters will claim that these colloidal supplements are "more natural" because they were taken from once-living plants that drew the minerals from the soil and are somehow "more balanced" because they contain so many minerals. Bull. The FDA has tested these products and found that colloidal minerals are not superior to any other source of minerals or in the most elemental form; i.e., in its simplest chemical structure. Using the word "colloidal" is hype, pure and simple.

And, of course, the ad includes a whole bunch of indefinite-as-to-quantity, unsubstantiated health claims.

If you get on the Internet and type in http://nature.webshed. com, you'll see a home page that presents an alphabetized box at the upper left-hand side. If you click on the "M" (which I did, just to see what they had for "Minerals"), you'll be transported to a rather incredulous destination. Just look at the following two ads. The first is for a product called "Mega-Chel."[2] Look at the amounts of nutrients for just the vitamins. It shows vitamin A (beta-carotene) as being "40,000 IU/800%" of the USRDA. Recall in the previous chapter that the USRDA is basically a defunct measure. However, if you look at the table I constructed on page 93, it shows the Upper Limit—the DO NOT EXCEED LIMIT—that the amount for vitamin A (beta-carotene) is only 15,000 IU. This Mega-Chel is *over 300 percent higher than the Upper Limit!* Vitamin B_1 (thiamine) is almost 3,000 percent (30 times) higher! Vitamin B_{12} is approximately 800 percent higher!

The next product under "M" that I present is called "Monthly Maintenance."[3] That shows, for example, that the amount of vitamin E is 300 percent higher than the Upper Limit on my chart. Vitamin B_6 is 600 percent higher.

For both products, you can see for yourself how many vitamins exceed both the "Acceptable Range" and the "Upper Limit." I will give you the same type of chart for minerals later in this chapter. Look at

Mega-Chel [Circulatory] is a key product for the circulatory
system. It contains a large array of nutrients to support the entire
circulatory system-arteries, veins, capillaries and the tissues and organs
they service. For example, the combination contains vitamins C and B6,
demonstrated to reduce platelet adhesion and aggregation. Every 12
tablets provide the following:

	Amount	%USRDA
Vitamin A (fish oils and beta-carotene)	40,000 IU	800
Vitamin C	4,000 mg	6,664
Vitamin B1 (thiamine)	200 mg	13,333
Vitamin B2 (riboflavin)	50 mg	2,941
Niacin	100 mg	500
Calcium (chelated amino acid)	400 mg	40
Iron (ferrous gluconate)	10 mg	55
Vitamin D (from fish oils)	650 IU	163
Vitamin E	400 IU	1,333
Vitamin B6 (pyridoxine HCl)	150 mg	7,500
Folic acid	400 mcg	100
Vitamin B12 (cyanocobalamin)	250 mcg	4,166
Iodine (potassium iodide)	125 mcg	83
Magnesium (chelated amino acid)	400 mg	100
Zinc (zinc gluconate)	30 mg	200
Copper (copper gluconate)	250 mcg	12.5
Biotin	100 mcg	33
Pantothenic Acid (d-calcium pantothenate)	500 mg	5,000
Potassium (potassium citrate)	400 mg	*
Manganese (chelated amino acid)	5 mg	*
Selenium (chelated amino acid)	250 mcg	*
Chromium (chelated amino acid)	200 mcg	*

*USRDA not established
The formula also contains 1-cysteine HCl (750 mg), choline bitartrate
(725 mg), p-aminobenzoic acid (250 mg), 1-methionine (175 mg), citrus
bioflavonoids (125 mg), rutin (125 mg), adrenal substances (50 mg),
spleen substances (50 mg), thymus substances (50 mg), inositol (40 mg),
ginkgo biloba leaves (30 mg), hawthorn berries (25 mg) and coenzyme
Q10 (10 mg). Each tablet is yeast-free and contains natural forms of the
above nutrients for higher assimilation. *Take six tablets with meals twice
daily. (Also see Key Products)*

Stock No. 1611-1 (180)
Price: $41.40 Qty: 1   Add To Shopping Cart

View Shopping Cart   Empty Shopping Cart

that and then compare those amounts with the amounts given for Mega-Chel and Monthly Maintenance and ask yourself if you would feel safe taking those dramatically higher amounts.

*   *   *

If you think you're being overwhelmed, you're right. I've said several times that there is an explosion of ads on the Internet. To prove my point, I entered "Vitamins and Minerals" on my search engine through my Internet Service Provider, Bellsouth. This was done on 12 September 1999. I include one of the pages,[4] which shows the fiftieth through sixtieth results, but note just above the first one shown on the page. It lists, "Now displaying 50–60 of 72481 results." *Over 72,000 links!* And you wonder why I wrote this book. Unless you know the principles contained in this book, you'd be a sacrificial lamb to the gods of greed when it comes to trying to analyze the ads and separate truth from everything else.

If you've had a sharp eye, you may also have noticed in some of the ads the word "chelate." Be careful with this one. The hucksters love it. In fact, there are dozens of books that specifically concern themselves with "chelation" or "chelation therapy," some of them are even written by M.D.s.

Here's why: Chelate comes from the Greek word *chele*, which means "claw." The ring structure of the metallic ions is combined much as a claw would grasp an object. The claw is an organic (meaning it contains carbon) chemical that is simply called EDTA, which is a jawbreaker for ethylenediaminetetraacetic. If you've got your false teeth in tight, you pronounce it "EH-thul-en-DIE-uh-mean-tet-rah-a-SEA-tick." Ions are simply particles that carry an electrical charge.

EDTA was first synthesized over sixty years ago in Germany, and works best at the body's pH blood level of 7.4, which is exactly normal. The term pH stands for *potential of hydrogen*, which is another way of saying whether something is predominately acidic (high number of hydrogen ions in the blood) or alkaline (low number of hydrogen ions in the blood). What all this means is that EDTA, which is water-soluble, chelates only metallic ions that are dissolved

Monthly Maintenance [Glandular] provides nutrients which may be especially beneficial just before and during a woman's monthly cycle. Many women are especially vulnerable to physical stresses such as poor nutrition, lack of rest and overwork. Consistent nutritional supplementation may be needed to resolve longstanding deficiencies. A daily intake of 18 capsules provides the following:

	Amount	%USRDA
Vitamin A (beta-carotene)	15,000 IU	300
Vitamin C	1,000 mg	1,600
Vitamin B1 (thiamine)	50 mg	3,300
Vitamin B2 (riboflavin)	50 mg	2,900
Niacinamide	50 mg	250
Calcium	150 mg	15
Iron	15 mg	83
Vitamin D (cholecalciferol)	400 IU	100
Vitamin E (d-alpha tocopherol)	600 IU	2,000
Vitamin B6 (pyridoxine)	300 mg	15,000
Folic Acid	200 mcg	50
Vitamin B12 (cyanocobalamin)	50 mcg	800
Iodine	150 mcg	100
Magnesium	300 mg	75
Zinc	25 mg	160
Copper	0.5 mg	25
Biotin	60 mcg	20
Pantothenic Acid	50 mg	500
Manganese	10 mg	*
Chromium	100 mcg	*
Selenium	25 mcg	*
Potassium	100 mg	*

*USRDA not established
Also included are choline (500 mg), inositol (500 mg), bioflavonoids (50 mg) and PABA (50 mg). All of the above is in a base of Chinese herbs: dong quai root, peony root, bupleurum root, hoelen plant, atractylodes rhizome, codonopsis root, alisma bark, licorice root, magnolia bark, ginger root, peppermint leaves, moutan root, gardenia fruit and cyperus rhizome. *Recommendation: Six capsules three times daily during the last 10 days of the menstrual cycle (i.e., 10 days before the onset of menstruation).*

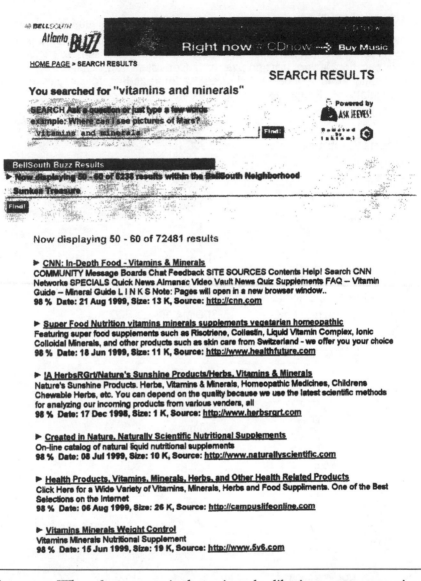

Now displaying 50 - 60 of 72481 results

▶ CNN: In-Depth Food - Vitamins & Minerals
COMMUNITY Message Boards Chat Feedback SITE SOURCES Contents Help! Search CNN
Networks SPECIALS Quick News Almanac Video Vault News Quiz Supplements FAQ – Vitamin
Guide – Mineral Guide L I N K S Note: Pages will open in a new browser window..
98 % Date: 21 Aug 1999, Size: 13 K, Source: http://cnn.com

▶ Super Food Nutrition vitamins minerals supplements vegetarian homeopathic
Featuring super food supplements such as Risotriene, Collestin, Liquid Vitamin Complex, Ionic
Colloidal Minerals, and other products such as skin care from Switzerland - we offer you your choice
98 % Date: 18 Jun 1999, Size: 11 K, Source: http://www.healthfuture.com

▶ IA HerbsRGrt/Nature's Sunshine Products/Herbs, Vitamins & Minerals
Nature's Sunshine Products. Herbs, Vitamins & Minerals, Homeopathic Medicines, Childrens
Chewable Herbs, etc. You can depend on the quality because we use the latest scientific methods
for analyzing our incoming products from various venders, all
98 % Date: 17 Dec 1998, Size: 1 K, Source: http://www.herbsrgrt.com

▶ Created in Nature, Naturally Scientific Nutritional Supplements
On-line catalog of natural liquid nutritional supplements
98 % Date: 08 Jul 1999, Size: 10 K, Source: http://www.naturallyscientific.com

▶ Health Products, Vitamins, Minerals, Herbs, and Other Health Related Products
Click Here for a Wide Variety of Vitamins, Minerals, Herbs and Food Suppliments. One of the Best
Selections on the Internet
98 % Date: 06 Aug 1999, Size: 26 K, Source: http://campuslifeonline.com

▶ Vitamins Minerals Weight Control
Vitamins Minerals Nutritional Supplement
98 % Date: 15 Jun 1999, Size: 19 K, Source: http://www.5v6.com

---

in water. What *that* means is that minerals, like iron, mercury, zinc, copper, calcium, etc., may be bound. If you're still with me, the hucksters have taken this somewhat complicated concept and turned it into another way to make money.

They claim that something that is chelated has better absorption, of course never telling you how much better or over what time period. What they don't tell you is that, while the minerals included in the formulas in their supplements may be better absorbed than the minerals that come directly from the foods you eat, what they don't tell you is that chelation increases absorption *and* excretion. *This means that the more you absorb the more you excrete, so there is no net gain!*

So you pay extra for something that works no better than what Mother Nature provides without human intervention. That's the expensive part. There is another part, and it has killed people.

This is chelation therapy, supposedly done to treat hardening of the arteries, blood poisoning, and mercury poisoning, and to be an alternative to coronary bypass surgery, among other claims (See Dr. Stephen Barrett's Quackwatch.com site). Simply stated, it is slow, intravenous infusion of EDTA and other substances. The treatment has been known to cost $75 to $125 per infusion, which is usually given one to three times a week, and each session lasts anywhere from three and a half to four hours. For a full exposition I direct you to the Web site http://www.quackwatch.com; scroll down to the article entitled "Chelation Therapy: Unproved Claims and Unsound Theories," by Dr. Saul Green.

I hope you're wondering what chelation therapy has to do with someone trying to peddle minerals to you. The answer is that, because those pushing chelation therapy have made such outlandish claims as to its benefits—none scientifically proven, by the way—the general public would "graft" or transfer the claims to the word "chelate" and then include it in the ads. What was hoped by the hucksters would be that the uneducated public would equate "chelate" with something scientific and beneficial and, therefore, desirable. The end result was supposed to be increased sales when the word "chelate" was used and/or misinformation about its benefits was presented. This is *exactly* what did happen.

The hucksters know that the vast majority of you are gullible and when they present you with something that is a little complicated they know you won't search for the truth—it's too much trouble. And that assumes you know something is *not* the truth. That's why they come on to you with the, "Oh, I'm so sincere and love all of you and want to help you and have the greatest thing here for you and please, because I'm such a wonderful and seemingly honest person, just give me your money (but whatever you do, don't challenge my statements or research my claims)." That's why a book like this is dangerous. It presents the truth. It's the one defense you have against their tactics. It costs them the amount of money you don't waste.

Athletes and people who consider themselves athletic may be some of the easiest marks for the hucksters, because we (I'm one of them) seem to be in a continual search for that "added competitive edge," or the latest scientific discovery that will make being in an athletic endeavor just a walk in the park—no effort, no pain, no sweat.

Take electrolytes, for example. These came to the forefront when various drinks, like Gatorade®, were invented. The concept was straightforward—you exert yourself, especially in hot and/or humid conditions and you'll sweat a lot. Do that, and your body will lose these precious things called electrolytes. For peak performance, your body needs to replace them.

Do you know what electrolytes are, and what they do? Electrolytes are minerals. There are three of them: sodium, potassium, and chlorine. They are dissolved in the body as ions (see above, for ions). These carry an electrical charge and are critical for the proper transport of nerve impulses in your neurological system, the stimulation/contraction of your muscles, and proper gland functioning. Sounds pretty important, doesn't it?

Well, they are important. I distinctly recall practicing and playing football in hot and humid conditions and remember players who had sweated profusely staggering around like they were drunk. Many collapsed. These sport drinks supposedly have solved that problem. That may be a true statement. What the hucksters don't tell you is that one eight-ounce glass of orange or tomato juice effectively replaces *all* the electrolytes lost in an amount equal to 7.04 *pounds* of sweat (that's 3.2 kilograms, for you metric fanatics).

Is 7.04 pounds of sweat a lot? Yes, it is. I learned early in my sports medicine training that only a 2 percent of body weight loss of sweat would result in dehydration. I weigh about 220 pounds. So 7.04 pounds of sweat would be 3.2 percent of my body weight, or more than 50 percent more than the amount that would result in my dehydration. The point here is that, while sports drinks work in general as advertised, their expense relative to the same volume of orange or tomato juice doesn't justify the expenditure.

The hucksters may also try and confuse you by labeling minerals as *major* or *minor* and try and attach some importance to that label. There are more than fifteen essential minerals. They *are* classified as major or minor (also called trace minerals).

Major or minor has *nothing* to do with importance. Major minerals are those whose minimum daily requirements exceed 100 mg per day. Minor minerals are those that are required in minimum amounts of less than 100 mg per day. If you added up all the milligram weights of minerals in your body, it would total about 15 grams or, for those of us who hate the metric system, about half an ounce.

The important *major* minerals are:

- Calcium
- Magnesium
- Phosphorus

The important *minor* minerals are:

- Chloride
- Chromium
- Copper
- Fluoride
- Iodine
- Iron
- Manganese
- Molybdenum
- Potassium
- Selenium
- Sodium
- Zinc

Here's what they do, as well as what can result from having too much or too little in your body. They are presented here, and in the table that follows, in the same order as I list them.

Calcium

Necessary for: Normal membrane permeability; activation of certain enzymes; (in salt form) the hardness and density of bones and teeth; (in ionic calcium in the blood and cells) transmission of nerve impulses, normal heart rhythm, and blood clotting.

Too much: Kidney stones; reduced functioning of the neurons in the nervous system; calcium deposits of salt in the body's soft tissues.

Too little: Retarded growth and rickets (abnormalities in developing shape and structure of bones) in children; osteoporosis, osteomalacia, and convulsions in adults.

Magnesium

Necessary for: Normal nerve and muscle excitation; conversion of adenosine triphosphate (ATP) to adenosine diphosphate (ADP) by acting as coenzyme constituent in the production of energy within the body's cells.

Too much: Diarrhea.

Too little: Tremors and neuromuscular problems; appears (as deficiency) in alcoholics and those suffering from severe kidney disease.

Phosphorous

Necessary for: Essential constituent of bones and teeth, proteins, nucleic acids, ATP, buffers of body fluids and phospholipids, which are necessary for the storage and transfer of energy, the activities of the nerves and muscles, and the permeability of the membranes of the cells.

Too much: No scientifically proven problems, though legitimate research has shown that an excess will reduce the absorption of iron and manganese.

Too little: Retarded growth and rickets.

Chloride

Necessary for: Transport of carbon dioxide (CO_2) in the blood; activation of salivary enzymes; pH balance of extracellular fluids, leading to formation of stomach acids.

Too much: Vomiting.

Too little: Severe diarrhea or vomiting leading to alkalosis (excessive alkalinity of body fluids); apathy; muscle cramps.

Chromium

Necessary for: Proper carbohydrate metabolism (especially by enhancing effectiveness of insulin); increases high-density lipoproteins (HDLs—they're the good cholesterol) and reduction of low-density lipoproteins (LDLs—they're the bad ones).

Too much: Not scientifically proven.

Too little: Not scientifically proven.

Copper

Necessary for: Manufacturing myelin, melanin, and parts of the electron transport chain; hemoglobin synthesis.

Too much: (Very rarely) Wilson's disease—characterized by tremors, muscular rigidity, spastic contractions, progressive weakness, emaciation, degenerative changes in the brain, cirrhosis of the liver, psychic disturbances, and dysphagia.

Too little: Extremely rare.

Fluoride

Necessary for: Strong tooth structure; prevention of dental cavities (especially in children); prevention of osteoporosis in adults.

Too much: Discoloring of teeth.

Too little: Unknown.

Iodine

Necessary for: Formation of thyroid hormones (T_3 and T_4) to regulate cell metabolism.

Too much: Depresses manufacture of the T_3 and T_4 hormones.

Too little: Shrinkage of the thyroid; goiter in adults; arrested physical and mental development (cretinism) in infants.

Iron

Necessary for: Binding of hemoglobin in oxygen transport system; proper functioning of oxidative phosphorylation (for energy creation).

Too much: Cirrhosis of the liver; heart and pancreas damage.

Too little: Anemia; constipation; flatulence; pallor of the skin; anorexia; paresthesias (heightened sensitivity to tingling, numbness, and prickling of the skin tissues).

Manganese

Necessary for: Normal kidney function; oxidation of carbohydrates and protein hydrolysis; interaction with enzymes to catalyze the manufacture of cholesterol, urea, hemoglobin, and fatty acids.

Too much: No known problems.

Too little: No known problems.

Molybdenum

Necessary for: Necessary constituent of various enzymes that aid in metabolism of nitrogen compounds found in coffee, fish, meat, and tea.

Too much: Leads to deficiency of copper; sharp pains in joints (similar to gout).

Too little: Not known.

Potassium

Necessary for: Effective transport of neural impulses, muscle contraction, glycogenesis and protein synthesis; maintaining correct intracellular membrane permeability.

Too much: Cardiac abnormalities, weakness of muscles, and paresthesias may result from severe alcoholism, kidney failure, and dehydration.

Too little: (Rare) heart failure; paralysis; vomiting; tachycardia; muscular weakness.

Selenium

Necessary for: Sparing of vitamin E; as an antioxidant; certain constituents of certain enzymes.

Too much: Fatigue; irritability; vomiting; nausea.

Too little: Not known.

Sodium

Necessary for: Acid-base balance in blood; normal neuromuscular function; pumping of glucose and other nutrients; maintaining osmotic pressure for extracellular fluid and water balance; maintenance of bicarbonate buffer system.

Too much: Hypertension; edema (swelling).

Too little: (Rare) muscle and abdominal cramps and nausea resulting from excessive vomiting, diarrhea, sweating, or inadequate dietary intake.

Zinc

Necessary for: Normal growth; sperm production; taste; smell; healing of wounds; proper carbon dioxide metabolism; constituency in several enzymes.

Too much: Tremors; slurred speech; walking difficulty; taut facial expressions.

Too little: Retardation of growth; loss of smell and taste.

As with vitamins, just because a mineral is necessary for something, it does not mean you need to take it as a supplement. Also, as with vitamins, keep a monthly log of everything you eat and drink. At the end of the thirty-day period, go back and compute your total intake and divide by thirty and add the totals to the first column (Minimum Requirement). If the sum of those numbers falls anywhere within the amounts in the second column (Acceptable Range), you probably don't need to add any to your diet. But keep in mind the risks for women that I have stated earlier in this chapter. Always consult your physician if you are in doubt as to whether you need to increase or decrease your intake. Don't self-prescribe and don't waste your money on hucksters.

Now I want you to have a little fun and be creative. Go back to the list of the minerals. Look only at the items following each mineral's "Necessary for" heading. What I want you to do is try and see if you can think of any grabbers or one-liners that could be used by hucksters to sell you that product. To get you started, just look at zinc. I wrote that it was necessary for sperm production, among others. Can't you see an ad, "INCREASE YOUR SEXUAL PROWESS! BE THE MAN YOU ONCE WERE! IMPROVE YOUR LOVE LIFE!" Go ahead and laugh. But not too hard. *Every one of those three phrases I just put in quotes was taken from* real *ads for products that contain zinc!*

Okay, now it's your turn, if you choose. If you do, treat yourself because you are learning how the enemy thinks—how they take a simple connection (like zinc-sperm production) and change it into money (yours) by extending the fact beyond reason. (By the way, zinc is not the only substance involved in sperm production. There are scores more.)

If you have done a real good job with your ads, you may find that you can spot a phony ad in the first few words, or, if you first see or hear it somewhere after the beginning, with just a few words. A trained ear, eye, and mind can shred the phony ads in no time with very little effort.

The table below provides the Minimum Requirement, Acceptable Range, and Upper Limit amounts for each of the essential minerals. The format follows that used for the table of vitamins.

Mineral	Minimum Requirement	Acceptable Range Low	High	Upper Limit
Calcium	150 mg	600 mg	1,800 mg	5,000 mg
Magnesium	125 mg	200 mg	600 mg	2,100 mg
Phosphorous	200 mg	500 mg	1,000 mg	3,500 mg
Chloride	90 mg	500 mg	1,000 mg	3,000 mg
Chromium	50 mcg	100 mcg	300 mcg	800 mcg
Copper	0.3 mg	1.0 mg	3 mg	10 mg
Fluoride	0.5 mg	2 mg	6 mg	20 mg
Iodine	30 mcg	100 mcg	225 mcg	750 mcg
Iron	5 mg	9 mg	27 mg	50 mg
Manganese	0.5 mg	1.2 mg	3.6 mg	12.5 mg
Molybdenum	20 mcg	50 mcg	200 mcg	750 mcg
Potassium	500 mg	1,750 mg	5,000 mg	15,000 mg
Selenium	10 mcg	35 mcg	100 mcg	500 mcg
Sodium	100 mg	250 mg	750 mg	2,000 mg
Zinc	2.0 mg	7.5 mg	22.5 mg	50 mg

Do you pay much attention to the nutrients listed on food labels? What I really want to call your attention to is the last few lines of the label. People often overlook it and they shouldn't, especially women. If you look at those last few lines it will usually give you the amounts of a few vitamins—usually A and C—and the amounts of some minerals—usually calcium and iron. Concerning minerals, I think I made a good case for their importance, especially for women. Don't jump the track and think the product in that container has that amount of calcium and iron in it. The amounts given are *per serving*. The amounts would only be the total in the container if the container held *exactly* one serving. But, if the container held four servings and the amount on the label said, "Iron 25%," that means that if you consumed all the food/drink in the container at one time, you'd be getting 100 percent of the *Daily Value* of iron. Note that most labels now list the nutrients (and amounts of fat, calories, etc.) in amounts and percents of the *Daily Value*. Go back to the previous chapter if you have forgotten what Daily Value means.

I will end this chapter with some interesting facts. Did you know that vitamins and minerals are not digested but released from the foods during digestion to be absorbed/excreted? Don't ever believe any ad that mentions the digestion of those nutrients.

The vitamin content of foods is determined by their genetic structure, not by the use of any kind of fertilizer. Some people think that fertilizers harm the vitamin content in foods. Baloney. This is the "all-natural" game again—making you believe any food grown with fertilizers is "not natural." Fertilizers *don't affect* the vitamin content of *foods!* Minerals in a food can be altered, but the difference is so small as to be irrelevant. Hucksters will try and convince you otherwise. Beware of the overused phrase "organically grown." The hucksters are lying to you if they say that plants grown with "natural" fertilizers, like manure, are more nutritious for you than those grown with synthetic fertilizers. That is not true. Each plant must convert any fertilizer—natural or synthetic—into the exact same chemicals before the plant can utilize them. Regardless of the type of fertilizer used, if there is one or more essential nutrients missing in the soil where the plant is located, the plant will simply not grow. It dies. No fertilizer can change that.

If a food is labeled as "organic," it is *not* any more nutritious (or safe for consumption) than any other food. The best "health-food" store you can find, and the best price you'll ever pay for health foods, is your local supermarket's fruit and vegetable section. All the rest is hype. Don't ever forget that.

Some hucksters try and dupe you by telling you that all diseases are caused by some deficiency in your diet. If you buy that line, then you're a sucker for the follow-on line which is, ". . . and, therefore, all diseases can be treated by an adjustment to your diet . . ." which usually leads right into the ad to tout their supplements. And it's all a lie. Where they try and snag you if you get resistant is to state that coronary heart disease (CHD) and osteoporosis are *caused* by bad diets. It is true that a diet high in cholesterol and low in calcium (especially for women) can *contribute* to CHD and osteoporosis, but to imply they are the sole cause is just pure bilge. But that's what the message is, and that's why you get duped.

Consider any food taken in moderation as a health food; any food taken in excess is junk food, regardless of the nutrients on the label.

Don't be a sucker and send a lock of hair away for analysis to determine the level of nutrients in your body. According to Dr.

Stephen Barrett's Quackwatch.com, no scientific study has ever proved this method of analysis to be effective.

Cooking, per se, does destroy to some degree vitamins and minerals in food. To minimize this loss, cook your foods in a microwave, if you can, with a quarter to one-half cup of water added, cover the container on/in which the food is cooked (if the instructions allow it), and eat all the liquid with the food. If you drain the liquid you cooked, you are throwing away some significant amount of vitamins and minerals.

Supplements should *never* be used as a substitute for foods, because foods contain literally *hundreds* of nutrients you can't get from supplements and your body knows better than any supplement manufacturer exactly how much of anything it needs at any point in time. Think about that. If you follow a trend line for the last fifty years, more and more supplement manufacturers are producing more and more products with more and more nutrients. Taken to its ultimate, logical conclusion, the manufacturers want to wind up literally producing synthetic food substitutes to entirely supplant your diet. And the cost to the consumer would be astronomical!

The most frightening thing is that it would be an extraordinarily unhealthy diet.

Nature has the perfect nutrition factory. Don't mess with it.

VIPS

Don't pay attention to the insipid ads that feature blinkers or flashers.

Minerals actually become part of the structure of the body (as calcium in teeth and bones).

To avoid the numerous and confusing interactions and counteractions of vitamins and minerals, don't take supplements (unless your physician directs). Let your body's natural physiology handle everything. It will do so automatically and optimally.

Women must be especially aware of likely deficiencies of iron and calcium.

The law allows anything to be claimed before a supplement is marketed and the FDA doesn't have the resources to pursue but a very few claims once the product has been marketed, even if the product harms you, makes you ill, or kills you.

Chelation adds no benefit to supplements because of the net gain of zero caused by increased excretion resulting from increased absorption.

"Sports drinks" may be fine but expensive. Drink one eight-ounce glass of orange or tomato juice and get the same benefits for a lot less money.

You only need fifteen essential minerals. Any product that advertises more is simply supplying you with something you don't need.

The next chapter sets the athletes and pseudo-athletes quivering. It has to do with all the so-called power supplements. The claims are basically, "Take this and you'll be stronger, faster, bigger, and healthier." Lot of "-er's" in there. They left out dumb-er and poor-er. You may even wind up dead.

NOTES

1. Montmorillonite. Internet advertisement printed from address http://www.vornet.com/~powerful/slmontmorillonitepage.html [12 September 1999], p. 1 of 2.

2. Mega-Chel. Internet advertisement printed from address http://nature.webshed.com/m-list.htm [19 September 1999], pp. 3–4 of 13.

3. Monthly Maintenance. Ibid., p. 9 of 13.

4. "Vitamins and Minerals." From Bellsouth search engine at address http://buzz.bellsouth.net/cgi-bin/gx.cgi/AppLogic+SearchPageAppLogic [12 September 1999], p. 1 of 2.

6

ERGOGENIC SUPPLEMENTS
A Lucrative New Class of Potential Killers

The kid looked terrible. He was a living, ten-year-old version of "Lurch," the monstrosity who was a character on the old *Addams Family* TV series. The kid had diabetes. His hands and feet were abnormally large. The bones and tissues in his face were also abnormally enlarged, making him look truly grotesque.

I said, "Son, where did you get the stuff?"

He replied, "Some guys at school sold it to me."

I queried, "Why did you take it?"

Calmly, he responded, "So I could look good for the girls."

His mother had brought the youngster into my sports medicine center. What the kid had taken was synthesized HGH—Human Growth Hormone. He had an advanced case of acromegaly (also known as Marie's disease). Acromegaly is a chronic disease of middle-aged persons characterized by elongation and unusual enlargement of head and facial bones, nose, jaw, lips, hands, and feet. It can also be caused by excessive HGH in younger persons. The person looks grotesque, like "Lurch." Acromegaly is *not* reversible. He would go through life looking like some sort of mutant. I'm not sure how long that life would be. Every day he looked in the mirror, he'd see this ugly, malformed face staring back at him. My God! He was only ten years old! And he was already so concerned about "looking good for the girls" that he became a tragic sucker.

HGH is produced naturally by the pituitary gland. Until about fifteen years ago, the only way to get extra HGH was to freeze-extract it from a cadaver. It was used clinically for patients who suffered from retarded physical growth—dwarfism. That was a legitimate application. Then somebody was able to synthesize it in a lab. It quickly found its way onto the "streets" and it started a huge black market supply for anybody who wanted to get big and strong, or "to look good for the girls." No one told the poor devils who bought the stuff that there were potentially deadly side effects. In addition to the abnormal enlargement of the extremities of the body, there are diabetes, visual impairment leading to blindness, muscular weakness leading to immobility, and death.

HGH is in a class of what are called "ergogenic supplements." In the scientific community and literature, ergogenic supplements are also known as "ergogenic aids" and "sports ergogenics." As they relate to this book, there are subdivisions within those labels, such as physiological sports ergogenics and pharmacological sports ergogenics. To keep everything as simple as possible, I'll just use the term "ergogenics" to be all-inclusive.

Ergogenics are substances that are supposed to help athletes enhance their athletic performance by increasing the athlete's physical power (energy production). In a nutshell, ergogenics are supposed to make you bigger, stronger, and faster.

In some cases, the ergogenics are produced naturally in the body—such as with HGH. There are other ergogenics that are found in the body—such as creatine—but are *not* produced naturally by the body. They are created *from other substances* within the body. However, what some manufacturers have done is create the ergogenics outside the body by synthesizing them, so they can sell them to you to introduce back into the body to supplement what is already there.

Greed, ego, and insecurity are the prime motives in the quest for improvement of human performance where ergogenics are involved.

Sport has become an enormously lucrative business. Literally millions of people want a piece of the pie, whether the pieces are named agent commissions, salaries, bonuses, ownership, memorabilia, apparel, speaking fees, endorsements, equipment, exercise apparatuses, magazines, papers, books, talk shows, betting services, prescription and nonprescription drugs, and substances (like ergogenics) and . . . well, the list goes on and on. The desire seems to be insatiable. When I see some illiterate jock say, "Well, I mean, y'know, I was offered, y'know, $4 million a year, and I had to, y'know, like, I mean, had to do what's best for my family, y'know, so I had to hold out for $5 million a year, because, like, I mean, it wasn't the money, y'know, it was respect, y'know, and I just couldn't accept only $4 million a year." Y'know? It's greed, you idiot. Why don't you have the guts to admit it? When I think of women, for example, who might have to spend their whole life in some dead-end secretarial job, trying to support a family, and not make $4 million in their *whole lifetime*, and that illiterate jock just can't make it on $4 million a year, I want to throw up.

The ego is a deranged, transfer association. The "I" has become the collective "we," such as in, "*We* are Number One," "*We* won the Super Bowl," "*We* beat the hell outta you guys." No, *you* are not Number One, *you* did not win the Super Bowl, and *you* did not beat the hell outta anybody. A team did. A team which you do *not* own. It's *not* your team. You are *not* a team member. You may be a fan of the team. That's all you are. (This doesn't apply to Green Bay packer fans—the Packers are a *publicly* owned team.) There is no transfer of performance from the team to you. Get it straight.

The insecurity is a curious dichotomy of the mind-set. Here we have athletes and pseudo-athletes who, for all their natural prowess are always looking for an additional "edge." Too many of them don't care how they get it. They simply refuse to accept their natural talents—and limitations—and look to science to provide the edge. If they just get completely orgasmic over all the things advertised as "natural," why is it that they continually seek that which is *not* "natural?"

The hucksters are smart enough to couch their advertising approach so as to avoid any connection with these drivers. They speak to alleged *results*. Where they include cautionary statements as to potential side effects (you almost never see them in the correct posture— *dangers*), the cautionary statements are for legal, not marketing, purposes. They don't want to get sued in their pursuit of your money.

The ignorance or boldness—or perhaps both—of the hucksters is truly amazing. In all honesty, I don't know how some of the people who create ads do so. What they say is so untrue, one would think their ad would result in more trouble than money, and they would opt to not publish an ad.

However, due to the money and notoriety associated with sport, it appears that this is the arena, more than any other, where we see the truly bold and stupid ads. As an example, I offer you the ad (below). Truly deserving of an award.

If I had to put money on an ad getting yanked, here's where I would place my bet. It's an ad for DHEA[1] (which I'll explain below). I want you to focus on the third paragraph, where I circled a phrase and noted my reaction ("BS!") next to it. The phrase is ". . . converting fat to muscle." Ladies and gentlemen, I will be brief and forceful: *Fat is not muscle. Muscle is not fat. Fat can never be converted to muscle. Muscle can never be converted to fat. Period. No exceptions.*

If I could sit you at a table with an electron microscope, and have you view fat and muscle, you would see they are entirely different. The anatomy (how they are constructed) and physiology (how they function; that is, how they react to things and how they work) are entirely different. If you had an eternity to sit at that microscope, you could bombard those two substances with an infinite number of other substances and the fat would never be converted into muscle and muscle would never be converted into fat. *Never.*

Now look at the second paragraph. I want you to notice the relationship of DHEA levels to age that are presented. This ad is way off the mark. First, most of us will not live to be age eighty. The maximum life span for females in the United States is 79.3 years and 75.6 years for males. Yeah, I'd say DHEA levels at age eighty would be a lot less than what we had in our twenties. Most of us are dead before age eighty. That'll really cut down the level.

Additionally, I personally researched DHEA levels of males and females in this country. How this was done is fully explained in chapter 14 on aging. More than 200,000 scores showed the DHEA levels at age seventy-five, when compared to age twenty-one, was 6.8 mcg/ml (micrograms per milliliter) and 0.8 for females, and 7.1

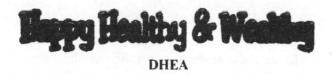

DHEA

DHEA is called the mother of hormones by researchers because it is used by the body to manufacture many other hormones, including our sex hormones that are necessary for many body functions. Some of these are well known, such as estrogen, testosterone, progesterone, cortisone and others. They are responsible for the maintenance of many body functions such as fat and mineral metabolism, controlling stress, maintaining male and female characteristics and others. The body produces DHEA and then converts it on demand to these other hormones. In addition, it is said that each of our cells also have DHEA receptors, meaning that DHEA has its own effects as well.

This wonderful substance is abundant in our bodies when we are about 20 years old but continues to decrease with time. At 80 years of age, we usually only produce 10 to 20% of the amounts when we were in our 20's. Interestingly, the steady declining levels of DHEA in our blood stream as we age perfectly matches the increasing incidence of the killer diseases cancer, heart disease (including atherosclerosis) and Alzheimer's disease.

One of the most exciting benefits of DHEA is its ability to burn fat and help keep it off by converting fat to muscle. It is a "thermogenic" substance because it helps burn calories for energy rather than store them as fat.

New studies have also pointed to the possibilty that DHEA supplementation may slow down the "aging process" by increasing overall energy and restoring memory.

Is DHEA right for you? Ask your doctor! .The best way to determine your DHEA dosage is to get your DHEA levels checked through blood or saliva tests - in fact, those under the age of 40 should have their DHEA levels checked prior to taking it, because you may not need DHEA supplementation. But for those of us over forty, it may be "just what the doctor ordered" when it comes to feeling younger!

Certain people should avoid DHEA. Women who are pregnant, nursing or thinking they may become pregnant, should avoid DHEA.You should also avoid DHEA if you are taking regular aspirin or blood thinners, stimulants (including herbs) or thyroid medications. If you are taking estrogen therapy, it is recommended to contact a physician to have your DHEA and estrogen levels tested.

Suggested Use: One to two tablets three times per day.
(Reference 1)

FOUNTAIN OF INFORMATION
CATALOG EMAIL US

and 0.4 for males. That is not, as the ad says, ". . . 10 to 20%. . . ." In fact, it works out to be 13.11 percent for females and only 5.63 percent for males. And this was from ages twenty-one to seventy-five, not eighty. In fact, the scientific literature is almost totally void figures for either gender beyond age seventy-five.

I do subscribe to an excellent healthcare information service called *Intelihealth* brought to us by the great people at Johns Hopkins Medical School, an entity for which I have the highest respect. In a 28 July 1998 report, they stated, "Production of DHEA . . . dwindles to about 5 to 10 percent of its peak level by the age of 80." That report does state that there is some solid evidence that there is a rise in the level of prostrate cancer in men and breast cancer in women when DHEA supplements are used.

Before you jump on my head for not including the who/how many/when, etc. components of the studies, know that they were not stated in the report. However, I want you to compare what the hucksters say with what the physicians tell us. The hucksters are straining mightily to move you emotionally; to fill their ads with lies, partial truths, unsubstantiated evidence, and inference to get you to spend your money. The physicians are just the opposite. They tell you the evidence is not conclusive; more research needs to be done; there are dangers in the use of (whatever); they cannot, at this time, recommend something's use. One group wants your money. The other group wants you *not* to be harmed. To which group are you going to listen?

What is repulsive is that the producer of this ad has probably made money as a direct result of what is stated in the ad. I do not care one iota that the ad has disclaimers or cautions. The essence of the ad is a lie. It is false. It is not true. So, Happy Healthy & Wealthy, whoever you are, may your ad sink in the cesspool of falsehoods with the rest of the crap being foisted upon the innocent public.

That ad refers to DHEA, which is shorthand for dehydroepiandrosterone (dee-HI-dro-ep-ee-an-DROSS-tear-own). DHEA is a steroid hormone produced naturally in your body by the adrenal gland. Even with all the hundreds of studies that have been done that include DHEA, we still are not exactly sure of all the functions it performs in the human body. For that reason alone, it should never be taken unless directed by a physician.

What DHEA appears—I said *appears*, *not* 100 percent proven to happen every time—to do is to be converted into other hormones, such as testosterone and estrogen, among others. It also appears to increase the level of IGF-I (insulin-like growth factor I), which is an anabolic (growth/building) substance that is *associated with HGH secretion*. That's the same HGH that I highlighted at the beginning of this chapter.

What the hucksters do is say that DHEA has been clinically proven to build bigger and stronger muscles and reduce fat. That's not the whole truth. I've read those studies. Some of the studies were done on rats, not humans. The DHEA level of rats is relatively much lower than humans across all comparative age groups. So, when a living organism that naturally has a low level of DHEA is given it as a supplement, you naturally expect significant results. That's exactly what happened—to the rats, not the humans.

Other ads will say that the studies were done on humans. Again, only the partial truth is presented, because the humans studied were all sedentary. So one would logically expect an improvement when the subjects were couch potatoes to begin with.

Ah, say the hucksters, but what about the subjects who were not rats or couch potatoes? What about them? They got no larger/slimmer. They *perceived* themselves to have larger muscles and less body fat, but the physical measurements did *not* show it to be true.

A new scam has arisen. Some people are promoting a Mexican yam (Discoria—also spelled "discorea"—the word, whichever way it's spelled, is the species of yam). They say that this yam is actually the "building blocks" for DHEA and that this yam is converted into DHEA once it is ingested into the body. (By the way, the process of ingesting something into the body and then having the body convert it to something else is said to be a "precursor" of something; that is, it precedes it.) This yam does contain a plant sterol ring that is used in the semisynthetic production of DHEA (and some other steroid hormones), this conversion can take place *only* in the laboratory. It is *not* a natural process as the hucksters want you to believe. The hucksters would also want you to believe that discoria can not only increase the body's production of DHEA, but also of testosterone and progesterone. Not true!

But the hucksters of discoria don't tell you the whole story. Here's the rest of it. Not too many years ago the only source of steroid hormones was from the glands of animals, but it wasn't easy and it wasn't cheap. It took something like 1,300 pounds of ovaries from some 50,000 sows to get only 20 mg of pure crystalline proges-terone. It was soon discovered that the principal raw material for, of all things, birth control pills was, of all things, discoria!

So the hucksters thought it would be a neat marketing trick to connect a woman's postmenopausal lack of estrogen with the yam. So they started peddling the yam as a way not to have to take estrogen and they also promised that it would increase a woman's level of DHEA, never once warning about the dangers of messing around with hormone levels in the body.

Just a couple of years ago, a laboratory said that some of the Mex-ican yam-containing products didn't contain or act as precursors to DHEA or progesterone. Well, that was certainly nice to hear. But, if that's true, why are the hucksters still marketing that yam product *as if it still did?* What, and whom, are we to believe?

The FDA never premarkets tests or evaluates premarket claims. The 1994 Dietary Supplements Health and Education Act (DSHEA) didn't change that. Federal law requires all new drugs be approved before marketing. The marketing of DHEA is supposed to be illegal, but the FDA has not enforced the law. This is some evidence that DHEA is not a "hot, new product." I've personally known of its exis-tence and use in sport for almost thirty years.

There is absolutely no scientific evidence whatsoever that the supplemental use of DHEA causes athletes to get bigger (bulk up), as the evidence shows no ability whatsoever of DHEA to act in anabolism (building up) or decreasing body fat. But, if you scan the ads—uncritically—you would think HGH and DHEA were the foun-tains of youth, the secret to longevity, the "pop a couple of these and you'll look like 'Ahhnold' in no time," and other such ludicrous claims. Know why those ads are so numerous? Because many people are get-ting duped, that's why.

In case you're wondering—yes, there have been deaths reported from the use and abuse (taking more than the label recommends) of DHEA and HGH supplements. But why should a few dead bodies concern the hucksters? There's so much money to be made from the suckers!

The list could go on and on, but I know the best reaction would be for the manufacturer and/or ad maker to tell the whole truth, not to take a partial truth and present it as the ultimate, uncontestable, all-encompassing truth. Put the burden of proof on them. This won't happen until you, the consumer, stop buying their product. I am not going to spend hours analyzing every ad that comes along. In fact, I have become so proficient at spotting the phonies (which includes just about everybody), I wouldn't pay any attention to them, save for including them in this book.

You, the reader, can become just as proficient as I am. It doesn't take a whole lot of practice, but it does take *some* practice. You'll know you've reached the big leagues when you can spot the lies, misrepresentations, mistakes, and come-ons as they occur. For example, if you were reading the Happy Healthy & Wealthy ad and you came to the phrase I highlighted and immediately you knew the ad was worthless, you would be in the big leagues, a force to be reckoned with, a sucker no longer. You would have power, because you know the truth.

You don't owe the hucksters your time. You don't owe them your attention. You don't owe them your effort to find some redeeming quality in their ad. You don't owe them your loyalty. You can give them some things, however. You can give them your scorn. You can give them your rejection. You can laugh at their futile attempts to take your money. You have better things to do, I'm sure, with your life than sit around just waiting to be duped.

If you really want to brighten up your life, do what my friends and I do. Here's the scenario: I'll have some people over for dinner. When dinner is over, we retire to the TV room and turn on the set and surf through the cable channels until we come to someone spewing the typical BS. As soon as they come to a "choker," we hoot and holler and shout deserved scorn. A "choker" is a point in the ad that stops the truth. It only takes a few seconds. For example, if what was being said was, "This product is incredible (choker— "Awww, BS!" "Forget it!" "Baloney!") and guaranteed to melt those pounds right off. . . ." I'm sure you get the idea. What is so unusual is that we seem to always be able to find some channel that is playing one of these ads. Some go on for a full half hour. And, if you switch channels, *you see that very same ad on another channel*. I will say that our evenings are filled with raucous laughter, good times, a lot of bonding, and the realization of how quickly—and how many times—an ad will hit a choker. Enjoy.

But don't turn on your TV set just yet. Look at the next ad, one simply entitled "DHEA," from some entity called "lifelink" (at least by the Internet address).[2] If you look at the items I circled, you will quickly discover ". . . the most recent paper studied . . ." is never named. Typical. And that paper supposedly states: "DHEA will improve the quality of life . . . and . . ." Hold it right there! We are never told what those quality-of-life components are or how they are measured. When the word "and" is placed in that sentence, it separates ". . . fatigue and muscle weakness" from the portion of the sentence referring to the "quality of life." We are not told why, how—or even if—the ". . . European pharmaceutical specifications . . ." are better (more stringent as to quality, potency, content, and absorption), equal to, or worse than U.S. standards. You could see this coming. Under "Key Benefits" the quantity is never mentioned; the measuring device(s) and methodologies are not stated; the group(s) of individuals who composed the stud(y/ies) are not identified nor is it stated how they were selected; the animals whose life span was supposedly extended are not identified; and . . . oh, you get the idea. There is absolutely no evidence that the information presented was derived by the scientific method.

It seems that the Internet is fast becoming a theme park for peddlers of disinformation.

Another ergogenic is chromium picolinate (we refer to it as "c-pic'" or "chromium pic'"). The big marketing campaign as I write this chapter (September 1999) is to tie chromium with chromium pic'. Here's why: Chromium is having some astounding sales success because it's touted to burn fat and build muscle (none of it scientifically proven, of course, but why let that little problem stop them?). You may not see chromium per se advertised as this "miracle," but rather chromium pic'. Why? Chromium normally acts *outside* the cell. Combine chromium with picolinate (which is an organic sub-

DHEA

[handwritten: name it] *[handwritten: By whom]*

DHEA (dehydroepiandrosterone) is a naturally occurring androgen, produced by the adrenal glands and is abundantly found in plasma and brain tissue. At the age of 21, we produce the highest levels of **DHEA** but by the time we reach age 40, our **DHEA** production plummets to half of that. Researchers contend that **DHEA** is the most significant endocrine bio-marker known, and further postulate that all of its effects may be explained by its action as a precursor hormone to estrogen, androstenedione and testosterone. There have been over 2,500 published papers documenting **DHEA's** multiple benefits, but the most recent paper studied the quality of life using this natural hormone: "**DHEA will improve the quality of life over a longer period and will postpone some of the unpleasant effects of aging, such as fatigue and muscle weakness.**" LifeLink's **UltraPure** brand is the only DHEA manufactured to European pharmaceutical specifications. The **UltraPure** brand of Micronized DHEA should not be confused with other DHEA products because our **Micronized DHEA** is 2-3 times more bioavailable than the standard form.

Key Benefits

[handwritten: better or worse than U.S? what are they]

- Support Healthy cardiovascular function
- Boost energy production
- Promote healthy mental function
- Enhance your body's natural immune response
- Improved sense of well-being
- Increases libido
- Extended lifespan in animals
- Decreased fat
- Reduced Stress

What is DHEA?

Micronized VS Standard DHEA

DHEA vs Lupus

Pricing

---

stance), the end product—chromium pic'—usually can work its way *inside* the cell to the very nucleus of the cell because the chromium pic' has a higher level of cellular absorption. It's terribly important that it get to the nucleus of the cell because this is where the "command center" of the cell is located and, in fact, where the chromosomes are located.

So, what's the big deal? Well, there are several deals. The first is there is no scientific evidence that chromium or chromium pic' burns fat. There is no scientific evidence that chromium or chromium pic' builds muscle. There *is* evidence, from test tubes and animal studies done in laboratories, that chromium has caused cells to mutate and begin to reproduce without limit. You know what that is called? It's called "cancer." Cells go out of control and their "command center" sends out only one message: "Reproduce. Reproduce. Reproduce . . ."

I admit, there is no evidence that chromium pic' will cause cancer in humans, but this may never happen. Why? *Because no reputable agency or foundation is going to fund a study to deliberately try and harm the patient by seeing if something can cause cancer in their bodies.* You would do well to read that sentence again. Hucksters will dupe you by saying, "Oh, this product has never been shown to cause cancer in humans." The implication is that the product is safe. The reality is that no one knows for sure and, by taking the product, you are in the unenviable situation of being a human guinea pig for something that may kill you, usually slowly and painfully.

If you want to play it safe and you've calculated that you do need to increase your chromium intake, don't buy chromium pic'. Instead, buy some brewer's yeast, because it has chromium but not the picolinate.

If you see any ad for chromium pic' that claims it will:

- Build muscle;
- Reduce serum cholesterol;
- Treat/prevent diabetes;
- Cause weight loss;
- Regulate blood sugar/insulin levels;

just ignore the ad. The claims are all untrue and unproven.

But that is not going to stop the hucksters. Take a look at the following ad. This one comes to you via the Internet, at http://www. chromiumpicolinate.net/.[3]

Take a look at the second section, the one starting with, "My name is Trina Garrison." It says she was asked by her brother (who is not named, we have no proof the guy exists, whether he's beyond preschool, is a scientist, etc.) to tell her story. Do you believe she lost forty pounds in ninety days? That during that ninety-day period she did nothing different except take this "AM-300"?

She then presents a sentence that makes no sense. It begins with, "Believe me . . ." Then she states that, "Just about everyone I know that has or is taken AM-300 has lost weight or has benifited in another way." Just how many people do you know who have taken AM-300, Trina? What were their body weights before they took that product? How much weight was lost by each person, and please tell us the time period involved? What are these "other ways" that people "benifited"? The last section on the first page isn't much better.

You'll also note in that one section:

- "Chromium Picolinate" is capitalized, and should not be. It's not a proper name;
- "Im" does not contain an apostrophe. It should;
- This Trina says that this product is ". . . the only thing I could find that would work for me." She never says *what* she was looking for or what her problem is or was;
- She uses the word "taken." It should be "taking";
- The sentence that begins, "Just about . . ." has at least six errors in it and I can't figure whether that sentence ends after "dramaticaly!" or continues with the "&." If it's the latter, add three more errors to that one sentence.

You really wonder what kind of moron wrote that section. If your light's on in your attic and you know you can't spell, can't construct a single coherent sentence, know nothing of grammar or syntax, you get somebody else to write the section for you. Take your time. Just get it right. I ask you, dear readers, whether you would believe or trust with your health anyone who comes across as being as dumb as a fence post?

Take a look at the second page. See where it says "100% Risk Free"? After what I've presented on the previous couple of pages, do you believe chromium pic' is *risk free*?

Okay, former "dupees," I think you can see that this ad is chock-full of mistakes and unsubstantiated claims. Don't waste your money on the product or the person who would be on the receiving end of your money if you bought anything from such a ridiculous ad.

I think this is a good place to introduce some essential points of fact and clarification. They can serve as a trip wire to a phony ad. These points can apply to any ad.

WHAT IS *CHROMIUM PICOLINATE?*

Chromium Picolinate is an organic complex, a definite compound of
trivalent chromium and picolinate acid. This product has been patented
by the U.S. Department of Agriculture and is licensed under U.S. Patent 3,988.

Click Here now for Your free samples of
AM-300 with*Chromium Picolinate!*

My name is Trina Garrison,
I was asked by my brother to tell my AM300 success story.
So here goes.

AM-300 with Chromium Picolinate! Wow, what a great product!
So far I have lost 40 lbs in only 90 days.
Im just about where I need to be.
This is the only thing I could find that would work for me.
Believe me, I tried every thing, Doctors included & the
diets they put me on! Just about everyone I know
that has, or is taken AM-300 has lost weight, or has benifited in another way,
such as, My stepdad's blood pressure dropped dramaticaly! & Also we all felt
great while losing the unwanted pounds, which is what I like the most about AM-300.

I was introduced to this product by a close friend who was having,
& is still having great success with them the AM-300.
Not only is she losing lbs, but helping others lose weight as well.
While doing this, she is also earning an additional income! I would
like to say Thanks to her again & again for hooking me up with something that works!
AM-300 has truly changed the way I look & feel.
You will feel great as you lose the weight. Don't take my word for it, try

1. Totally disregard the "testimonials" (as you saw in the ad above). If
the testimonials were true, it would only be because enough
people had taken the product(s) in a scientifically controlled
study, and the results had been published and had stood the test
of professional scrutiny. You'll never see hucksters do this. They
won't do it because: (a) they have created a phony testimonial;
and/or (b) their product(s) will not work as advertised.

it yourself for 30 days and don't forget to let me know how it goes :)
Trina from Oklahoma, email

Give <u>AM-300</u> Natural Herbal Energizer with Chromium Picolinate
A honest try, & if not completely satisfied, return the remaining bottle for a full refund!
You have nothing to lose but those unwanted pounds and inches!

100% Risk Free!
AMS 30 day money back guarantee.

<u>Click here to see pic's & receive</u> Free Samples Of
*AM-300 **with** <u>Chromium Picolinate</u>*

<u>*AM-300 HomePage*</u>

For more info: Call (580) 255-1617
Toll Free 1 (877) 255-1617

Chromium Picolinate ▼

Go Get It!

Home

2. You see an ad that offers a free or low-cost health analysis just by filling out a simple questionnaire (oftentimes used to sell supplements). I've even seen them on computers in health spas. What a joke they are. If you want a true health analysis, see your physician. Filling out that questionnaire is risky, at best. Why? Take a look at what happened to yours truly. I was at a Gold's Gym in Alabama in 1997, where I sat down at their computer and the questionnaire came up on the screen. It asked eight general

questions, plus the estimated amounts of all the vitamins and minerals considered "necessary."

I deliberately entered more than *twice* the amount of vitamins and minerals any healthy person should ever need on a daily basis (at least twice the RDA). When I had entered the information and hit the "Enter" key, I waited about two seconds and voilà, my "Personalized Health Profile" showed on the screen. It presented that I was *deficient* in six vitamins and five minerals, and recommended I take DHEA, melatonin, and sawtooth palmetto!

Now it really gets interesting. A prompt on the screen told me I could order the "needed items right now!" on the computer. Just whip out my credit card. Or, I could order the stuff at the health bar in the gym. When I tried to print out my results, nothing happened. I was told I simply couldn't do it. The computer was not programmed to do it.

That's just outstanding. Somebody is trying to sucker me by creating a phony "Personalized Health Profile." I confronted the manager of the gym. To his credit, he said that somebody had sold them the software. He said they'd had so many complaints they were yanking it. He mentioned some people had even ordered what the computer told them to order, and never received the product(s). I checked back three weeks later. That computer software was gone. Good work, Gold's Gym.

The point is that, even though a questionnaire may appear to be a legitimate analytical tool, you can spot it as a fake if there is a purchase tied to the results. And the ads almost always result in you being "deficient" in some way or other, and it just so happens that the ad tells you that you can solve that problem right now by ordering some junk you most likely don't need. *Ignore these questionnaires entirely!*

3. Some ads will purport to be able to "cleanse your (body; a system—immune, digestive, reproductive, etc.—or even your mind)." *Don't believe them!* There is nothing—except good nutrition—that will cleanse your body of alleged "toxins" or "poisons" that the ads refer to, but usually never mention. Think about this: If you do have these unnamed "toxins" or "poisons" in your body, *why haven't they already killed you?* How long do you have to

live before these "toxins" or "poisons" do their number on you? How long will it take for the advertised products to "cleanse" you? I hope you see my point. If not, it is that your body already has a perfect system to clean itself out, if you'll just let it. Scare tactics and miracle promises are just a pack of lies. *Ignore such ads!*

* * *

Melatonin. The name has kind of a soft sound to it. It's pronounceable and not two hundred letters long, as some ergogenics seem to be. Its popularity seems to be lagging, but in the years 1995–1997 it apparently outsold even vitamin C. This gentle-sounding substance has some very powerful effects. Why the hype and what's the truth?

Melatonin is not an herb. It's not a "natural" food. It's a hormone produced by your body's pineal (pin-EE-al) gland (situated in the middle of your brain behind your eyes). It has been touted as a cancer preventive/cure, a sleep aid, an antiaging "medicinal" substance, a sex enhancer, and is claimed to calm erratic behavior and a host of other maladies.

The problem with melatonin is that it interacts with virtually every other hormone and scores of chemicals in the human body and we are not sure of all the reactions. We do know that its "safest" claim is as a sleep enhancer, especially where jet lag is concerned. What concerns me is that melatonin is not sold via prescription. Yet it is just as powerful a hormone as, say, testosterone. In fact, some melatonin (almost always produced from Europe) is not made synthetically, but is taken from the pineal glands of animals.

There is some scientific evidence that, in rats, melatonin acts as a powerful antioxidant and appears (not universally proven) to prevent some (not all) types of cancers and reduce (not destroy) some types of tumors. I don't like doing this. I don't like putting "qualifiers" in every sentence, especially when a lot of people are understandably nervous, scared, suffering, or merely inquisitive about something like cancer. But I feel honor bound to do so, because I believe a false hope is as bad as an overt lie. You should never take melatonin without your physician's prior approval, especially if you are under fourteen years of age; are pregnant; are nursing; or have any severe allergies, lupus, lymphoma, or any disease that is caused by a failure of your immune system.

As to claims that melatonin is a sex enhancer, antiaging "medicinal" substance, or a tranquilizer, according to the American Academy of Anti-Aging Medicine there is no scientific evidence that it does any of these things.

Boron was a hot item a few years ago. It was touted as having all the benefits of anabolic steroids without any of the dangerous side effects. Boron is not an ergogenic per se (as many are hormonal in nature) but a trace mineral being marketing as a powerful muscle stimulant, as well as a "bone grower" (i.e., some great substance that will hype the production of calcium in your body). Baloney. If you have, or think you have, osteoporosis, are postmenopausal, or are arthritic, you are especially targeted by the hucksters, because the claims of boron are (surprise!) made to make you believe boron can overcome all of these problems. The real problem is that almost every known malady in the human body is not—I repeat, *n-o-t*—the result of a deficiency of just *one* substance in the body. Therefore, increasing the amount of any one substance will *not* cure the problem. This is something the hucksters will never tell you.

As to boron's alleged effectiveness for the above-stated (and other) claims by the hucksters, they are almost entirely unproven, untrue, or misleading.

The newest fad (it's really an attack strategy) is to use only two words, such as "Osteoporosis. Calcium." "Sleep. Melatonin." "Anti-aging. HGH." "Arthritis. Boron." The whole idea is to get you to identify as having the first word (the problem; the need; the perception) and buy the second. What a crock! And it's potentially deadly. What the message is requiring you to do is self-diagnose (if you haven't had it medically determined previously) and then to self-prescribe. By shortening the "grabber" to only two words, the hucksters have opened the way for you to speak volumes. So you really dupe yourself big time, and it only took *two words* to get your money. I have two better words—please don't.

*   *   *

Androstenedione (an-drow-STEEN-die-own, and not "AN-druh-sten-eh-dee-OWN-ee, as someone on the Fox network called it while doing a story on Mark McGwire in 1998). Also known as "andro" by knowledgeable individuals as well as wanna-bes, its star may be fading. It exploded when Mark McGwire of the St. Louis Cardinals was consistently hitting monster home runs during the 1998 major-league baseball season. The supplement manufacturers almost got hernias loading all the bull into their ads for andro when McGwire said he used it. And they really loaded up on the amounts.

Here's what we know and what happened. Andro is included in the class of androgens, which are male sex steroids. Andro is a steroid which, in the adult body, is converted to testosterone and, in children (both boys and girls), it can also be converted into the female sex steroid, estrogen.

Andro is not found in our normal diet, so it cannot be treated as a "dietary supplement." We know that androgens can stunt growth, reduce sexual function, shrink the testicles, and shut off the normal production of testosterone.

Probably the most appropriate group to study andro is the Endocrine Society, which is the largest, most active, and oldest professional body that performs research on hormones and the clinical practice of endocrinology. What the society could not prove was everything the hucksters did use as claims, namely,

- Whether andro can enhance athletic performance;
- Whether taking andro is safe or effective;
- What andro's absorption rate is and, once in the body, where it goes;
- Whether or not it causes liver cancer like other androgens;
- What the purity of the commercially produced andro is.

The only thing that caused joy for the manufacturers was the society has not as yet been able to invent a test that can detect andro.

Don't take any substance like andro, which has so many detrimental side effects that are never mentioned by the hucksters. McGwire put a damper on andro when he announced at the beginning of the 1999 baseball season that he had stopped taking it and would not start up again. I'll wager some manufacturers were on their knees praying that Mark would have a lousy season so they could screech, "See! We told you! It was andro! That's the only reason he hit all those homers in '98!" In 1999 Mark hit *more* homers than he did in 1998, and he did it without andro. Sammy Sosa did the same thing.

I want to give credit where credit is due. Even though Mark makes a huge salary, I'm sure he could have made many additional millions if he would have given andro an endorsement. He never did, but instead gave credit to his years in the weight room, his batting coaches, the hitting background in Busch Stadium, starting to wear different contact lenses, the less dense air in St. Louis versus that in the San Francisco Bay Area (where he played for years with the Oakland Athletics), and—get this—eating a lot of natural, nutritious foods. Attaboy, Mark!

If I were giving a dual award, it would be shared by the manufacturer of the "Extreme Ripped Force (Thermogenic) Bar," American Body Building, and the people at the Web site http://getbig.com/abb/bar-rip.htm.[4]

I snicker at the site "getbig." You see, I'm not terribly impressed with some of the ingredients that are so easy to get in a normal diet. My problems with the ad are more with the name of the product—an infantile attempt to use the "action" words "extreme ripped force," and the disclaimer on the third page under "Warnings," where it states, ". . . heart attacks, stroke, seizure and death."

I really came unglued when I read that. I do not believe for a minute that the manufacturer or seller cares one bit for your health or life. Do you know why the exact words "Extreme Ripped Force" are in the product title? Do you know why anyone in their right mind would manufacture, advertise, or sell any product that could kill you if you simply took more than the one bar recommended? Why the hell are you putting your fellow human beings at risk, warnings or no warnings? Why not put the warnings at the very top of the ad instead of on the last page? Think little kids won't get hold of this "candy bar" and exceed the "recommended use"? Will some moron who thinks himself just too big physically say to himself, "I'm so big, I need at least two of these bars"?

I hope you readers have snapped to attention. Yes, some nonprescription products packaged as candy (bars) can kill you. If that doesn't make you want to read the entire label—warnings included—I don't know what will. The burden of proof in a wrongful death suit is not on the defendant. It's on the dead person's estate or whomever is acting as plaintiff in the suit.

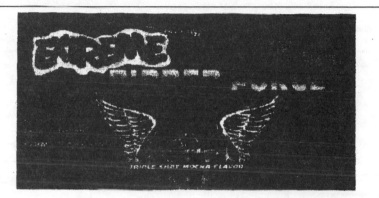

Extreme Ripped Force Bar!

The Description

American Body Building is excited to bring you their latest bar, the Extreme Ripped Force Thermogenic Bar. This bar is not for everyone. It is a powerful bar, the first of its kind, with 300mg of Ma Huang, 100mg Quercetin, and 150mg of Caffeine in it. This bar is designed as a preworkout bar, to increase energy, increase endurance, and maximize exercise intensity.

Take It To The

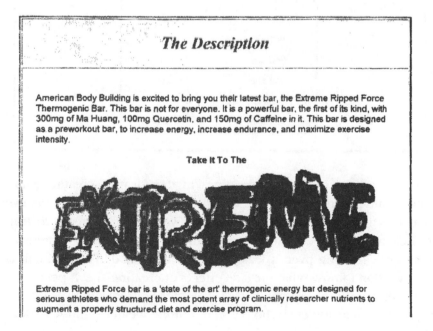

Extreme Ripped Force bar is a 'state of the art' thermogenic energy bar designed for serious athletes who demand the most potent array of clinically researcher nutrients to augment a properly structured diet and exercise program.

Benefits from Extreme Ripped Force's herbal ingredients include

- increased endurance
- Reduction of fatigue
- Improves reaction time
- Spares muscle glycogen
- Increases fat oxidation
- Enhances weight loss effects of diet and exercise.

Extreme Ripped Force bar currently comes in one flavor, Triple Shot Mocha!

The Facts

Serving Size	1 bar (45g / 1.6 oz)
Calories	160
Total Fat	3 g
Saturated Fat	2 g
Total Carbohydrate	33 g
Dietary Fiber	2 g
Sugars	11 g
Protein	3 g
Sodium	90 mg
Caffeine	150 mg
Ma Huang Extract	300 mg
Quercetin	100 mg

Two other ergogenics—creatine, in the form of creatine phosphate, and pregnenolone—are very popular. Right up front, I believe that creatine is effective in supplying a very small increase to lean muscle mass when used with a program of moderate to high intensive resistance training over at least a six-month period. The problem is that we don't know what the side effects of creatine are. It poses risk without benefit for everybody else. It's utter nonsense to use creatine if you are not an athlete, who is also not lifting weights, and who does

The Warnings

With a hyper-thermogenic performance bar this powerful, there are many warnings in which are important to know about. That is why we call it an Extreme!

Do not exceed recommended use. Taking more than the recommended dosage of one bar may increase the risk of side effects, which can include headaches, heart attacks, stroke, seizure and death. In other words, do not take more than one bottle.

Keep out of reach of children. It is not intended for use for people under the age of 18! In case of accidental overdose, contact a physician, emergency medical care facility or poison control center immediately.

Do not use if you are pregnant or nursing, or if you have high blood pressure, heart disease, diabetes, difficulty in urination due to prostate enlargement, or if taking a MAO inhibitor or any other prescription drug. Reduce or discontinue use if nervousness, tremor, sleeplessness, loss of appetite, or nausea occurs. This product is not intended to diagnose, treat, cure or prevent any disease. If you have other questions, seek the advice of a physician prior to using this product.

The Ingredients

Coating (Maltitol, Salatrim, Cocoa (processed with Alkali), Sodium Caseinate, Lecithin (as an emulsifier), Vanilla, Acesulfame-K), Corn Syrup, Rice Flour, High Fructose Corn Syrup, Whole Wheat, Milled Corn, Rolled Oats, Rice Bran, Sugar, Gellan Gum, Rolled Wheat, Barley Flakes, Natural and Artificial Flavors, Date Paste, Fig Paste, Raisin Juice Concentrate, Instant Coffee, Honey, Molasses, Malt Extract, Ma Huang Extract, Quercetin, Caffeine Citrate, Caffeine, Crystalline Fructose, Acacia Gum, Glycerine, Salt, Thiamin Hydrochloride, Pyrodoxine Hydrochloride, Niacinamide, Folic Acid, Calcium Panthotenate, Reduced Iron, and Zinc Oxide. The bar may also contain trace amounts of nuts or peanuts.

Back to the ABB Bar Menu

---

not first get approval from a physician. Why do I keep harping on getting your physician's approval? Because the products in this book have unknown side effects, the manufacturer does not know you or the health status of your body, and only your physician is skilled enough to know you and your body—specifically—to tell you "Yes" or "No" as to supplementation as well as "How much" and "How long," and what to do if you notice certain side effects.

Pregnenolone is really being touted as an "antiaging miracle." Don't you just love it? Miracles right in front of our eyes. And it only costs $12.95. Take a look at the ad for TriMedica's Pregnenolone.[5] They call it "an exciting breakthrough in anti-aging." It never says what the breakthrough is. Are you getting the idea that no ad is without omissions, lies, unsubstantiated claims, or missing facts (to name a few)? *Good.* That's the idea you *should* be getting. And the more you get it and can identify where the ad is faulty, the less of a susceptible consumer you will be to hucksters' ads.

Last, you should be aware of a whole class of supplements called "amino acids." Protein is made from amino acids. You can spot them because they usually end in "-ine." Examples are: ornithine, arginine, lysine, histidine, phenylalinine, and others. Note that while creatine is not in the previous list it is an amino acid because it belongs to a class of what are called branched-chain amino acids (BCAAs). Creatine is made from other amino acids, specifically, glycine, arginine, and methionine. Other BCAAs are leucine, isoleucine, and valine.

Quite simply, hucksters can't turn out enough ads for amino acids. Their rationale is that, since protein builds muscle, whatever builds protein is even more necessary. Since athletes are supposed to have larger muscles than the average person, the target market is the athlete. These days, anybody can buy anything (apparel) to fake it as a jock, so another market has developed and been targeted, that of the pseudo-jock, which seems at times to include most of us. So the ads keep getting more and more numerous. And the hucksters make more and more money.

As to amino acids and protein, your antenna need to be sharply tuned to the unfounded shouts of how much bigger, stronger, more muscular, less fat, and more coordinated you will be if you'll only take this pill or powder. Don't forget what I said at the beginning of this book. I have been duped many, many times. In fact, I remember taking protein in powdered form in late 1964, when I was a linebacker on the University of Notre Dame Freshman Football Team. During the next four years, in addition to weightlifting and running a lot, I tried anabolic steroids (once, for sixty days), and a forgotten amount of supplements. My undistinguished record on the gridiron should serve as moot testimony to the fake claims (or maybe I just wasn't that good).

TOLL-FREE ORDER LINE: 1-888-660-8831
QUESTIONS/PRODUCT INFO:
217-662-8831
EMAIL

PREGNENOLONE

Pregnenolone
50 ct, 30mg

An exciting breakthrough in anti-aging. Pregnenolone, a hormone produced by the adrenal glands. Unlike DHEA, which converts to estrogen and testosterone, Pregnenolone is converted directly to progesterone, and can be an excellent choice for estrogen- sensitive women or testosterone-sensitive men. Pregnenolone has been used for:

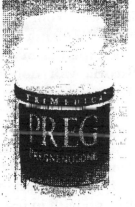

- PMS and menopausal problems
- Estrogen sensitivities
- Arthritis and fatigue
- Ovarian cysts

Product #1211 · Pregnenolone
30 ct/50 mg · $12.95
Case/12 · $114.00 ($9.50 ea.)

FAX ORDER FORM

For information about our return policy and guarantee, please **CLICK HERE**.

TO ORDER BOOKS ABOUT PREGNENOLONE, CLICK ON THE TITLE OF THE BOOK

My point here is that creatine phosphate (or any of the other supplements) in 1964 was the same as it is in 2001. The claims are more numerous. I don't recall anyone hyping antiaging, immune system function, or postmenopausal relief thirty-five years ago. Only the ads have changed. And more people have died because of them. The promised results have not, as a general rule, ever been achieved. But we continue to waste our money. We continue to be disappointed in the promised results.

VIPS

Stay away from HGH unless you have your physician's approval. If HGH results in acromegaly, it is *not* reversible.

Stay away from DHEA unless you have your physician's approval. We do not know all of the functions and changes it alters or produces in the human body.

Discoria will not increase your body's production of DHEA, testosterone, estrogen, or progesterone. And it will not cause you to have larger muscles.

If you need to take chromium, do so by taking wheat germ. Chromium pic' should never be used as a chromium supplement. Chromium pic' may cause cancer. It is not a scientifically proven weight-loss or muscle-building product.

Place no faith in testimonials, "health questionnaires" that are not part of an overall physical/health medical exam, or any product claiming to "cleanse" your system.

Do not take megadoses of any supplement without your physician's approval. Some instances of megadosing have caused the body's normal production of the supplement to shut off and not restart when the megadosing was halted.

Melatonin may be effective for jet-lag sleeplessness. In any case, take it only with your physician's approval.

Boron has never been scientifically proven to grow bones or muscles.

Creatine (in the form of creatine phosphate) has been scientifically proven to cause minimal increases in strength, but

only when coupled with weight-training programs of several months when used by athletes, and it has not been scientifically proven to benefit endurance athletes (like bike riders). The beneficial results have only been proven for "short burst" sports like weightlifting and football.

Ignore ads with just two words like "stop stress" or "lose fat." You will be self-diagnosing and self-prescribing if you take those products.

Andro has not been scientifically proven to enhance athletic performance, and we do not know if it is safe and effective, what its absorption rate is (and where in the body it goes), if it causes liver cancer in humans, or what the purity of commercially produced andro is. All we know is that we haven't found a test to detect various levels of it in humans.

Ignore any products with extreme wording, like "Ultra-Mega-Extreme Weight-Loss Powder," in the name of the product. It may kill you.

Pregnenolone has no scientifically proven antiaging properties.

Amino acids construct protein. There is no scientific evidence that they will make you bigger, stronger, faster, or give you better reflexes.

The next chapter is the great "grab bag." I name it so because it appears that if you have something wrong with you—anything—there is an herb, or combination of herbs, that will fix or cure anything that ails you. Nothing could be farther from the truth. And, to keep you off guard, the manufacturers include herbs with certain vitamins, minerals, ergogenics, and other supplements to supposedly enhance the results, all by some seeming "mystical, synergistic" properties. Adding all these ingredients can be overwhelming, unless you are learning that, if one product is ineffective as touted, and you add another ineffective product, one ineffective plus one ineffective does not equal one effective anything!

NOTES

1. Happy Healthy & Wealthy ad for DHEA. Internet advertisement printed from address: http://www.happyhealthyandwealthy.com/dhea.htm [6 May 1999], pp. 1–2 of 2.

2. Lifelinknet ad for DHEA. Internet advertisement printed from address: http://lifelinknet.com/dhea.htm [6 May 1999], p. 1 of 2.

3. Chromiumpicolinate ad for AM-300. Internet advertisement printed from address: http://chromiumpicolinate.net/ [6 May 1999], pp. 1–2 of 2.

4. Getbig ad for Extreme Ripped Force Bar. Internet advertisement printed from address: http://www.getbig.com/abb/bar-rip.htm [15 May 1999], pp. 1–3 of 3.

5. Holbrook ad for TriMedica Pregnenolone. Internet advertisement printed from address: http://www.holbrook.net66.com/~carla/sepregnen.html [6 May 1999], p. 1 of 2.

7   HERBAL SUPPLEMENTS
Can You Handle the Truth?

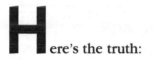ere's the truth:

- The manufacturers of herbal supplements and remedies do *not* have to prove the safety or effectiveness of their product
- Some herbs have been proven to possess limited and mild beneficial effects on certain nonlife-threatening conditions, but also have been proven deadly when used in combination with other drugs and/or supplements.
- No one knows for sure how many different herbs are on the market, singularly or in combination.
- There is no database, in any form (book, manual, computer database) that lists all known herbs and their real and potential interactions with prescription and nonprescription drugs.
- There is absolutely no guarantee whatsoever as to the content, quality, purity, and absorption of an herb, either individually or in combination with any other supplement(s).

If your vital signs are still on the chart, you've been around long enough to know that it seems you can pick a health problem—any health problem—and somebody out there has an herbal remedy to cure it. This image is not created by mistake. Your mistake is believing the image.

Herbs seem so . . . "nonoffensive," might be a good word. Yet, we know very little about them. As an example, here are some interesting factoids about an extremely popular herb, ginseng. There are several different kinds of ginseng, and even the same ginseng root can yield several different substances. Ginseng has several different names—ginseng, radix ginseng, ren-shen, and *Panax ginseng*. This naming is applied to both Siberian ginseng as well as oriental American ginseng. Do you have any idea of these differences? Did you ever take "ginseng" of any type and *know* what you were taking?

If the name game doesn't cause enough complications, when mixed with vitamins, minerals, and/or ergogenics, the picture becomes even more distorted. Whereas herbs are incorrectly given the status of "cures," the other three groups are more often considered "enhancers." Oh, the industry just loved that one. They effectively said, "Hey! If we combine cures with enhancers, can't we then market the combination as 'enhanced cures'?" People probably got trampled in the rush to the ad agencies and the Internet Web masters.

The essential question people ask is, "Well, are herbs effective cures or not?" You'll hate the honest answer: "Some do. Some don't." Before you bail out on me, let me explain. Those "health problems" that some herbs "cure" are all mild in nature. None that *do* act as cures have been scientifically proven to be 100 percent effective all the time. Some of them are deadly; they have killed people. So, the beneficial aspects are mild, at best, deadly, at worst. (See Dr. Stephen Barrett's Quackwatch.com.)

The curing, even when done, has been one of *degree*. There are *no known cases* of any herb curing a serious medical ailment all by itself. Not one. And this problem of degree is even further complicated if, say, your neighbor says, "Well, I took (whatever) and it worked for me." What is that supposed to mean? What kind of endorsement is that? Seriously, is that the *only* thing your neighbor took for the problem? How serious was the problem and who determined just how serious it was? Are your symptoms exactly the same as your neighbor's? How do you know that? How do you know that, even if you took the same herb, it would be the same as to purity, content, quality, and absorption? The answer to all those questions— if answered truthfully—would have to be: "I don't know."

The hucksters have added some power to herbs in the form of what they are being called—phytomedicinals. "Phyto-" is a Greek prefix that means "combining forms, or indicating a plant or something that grows." The "medicinal" base word is what is being emphasized and I see it as a two-edged sword. It may, in fact, make herbs seem more potent because of the not-very-hidden root word "medicine." It's as if their message is that herbs are medicine and you don't need a prescription. In fact, the hucksters will tell you that many countries use herbs as medicines far more than prescription medicines. That's true. Well, it's only half true. What you are *not* told is that those countries have such low personal incomes that the people can't afford the prescription drugs, and their high death rates prove it.

Oddly, these same hucksters will tell you some of the herbs come from the bark of a tree in some mysterious rain forest, though they never tell you where it is located.

Oftentimes, you will be duped by information—most often presented in pictorial or graphic form. That picture or graph is worth a thousand words (and a lot of sales). At least the hucksters hope it will be. It also is important enough to be stated as a principle.

☐ #11. THE PRINCIPLE OF THE STRAIGHT-EDGED TRUTH-STRETCHER

The Principle of the Straight-Edged Truth-Stretcher is the practice of presenting a picture or graph that does *not* show the results of a study, but the hucksters want you to believe it does. I love this one, especially in the context in which it is employed. In fact, it's such a graphic and suggestive one, I have a hard time typing and laughing at the same time. It is so good, it is deserving of an award. And this is not the first time that the company, Gero Vita International, has claimed the prize in this book. They seem to send me a flyer every month claiming to have a cure for one of the real pressing problems of our time.

Look at the following illustration. It is for a product called *Testerex*, from Gero Vita International.[1] The headline might be true, if you consider I don't get terribly "excited" about reading some of these ads. I'm going to ignore the other eleven pages of the flyer, because the content really is not relevant to my analysis. Just look at the graph and the paragraph underneath it. I ask you, doesn't that graph seem to go with that paragraph? The manufacturer sure hopes so, but if that is what you think, you've just been duped again.

Here's why: First, notice that each of the three lines—volume, length, and circumference—are all straight lines. Perfectly straight lines. In science, this represents what we call a "perfectly direct relationship," which means that there is *exactly* the same change relative to the horizontal axis (age) as there is for the vertical axis (percent). In other words, if you move, say, from age thirty to forty on the volume line, you'll get a specific change in the percent. In this case, it looks to be 3 percent, from 21 to 18 percent. Here's the kicker. If you move *any* ten years on the volume axis, you'll always get that 3 percent change. Try it. If you move from age twenty to thirty, the change in percent is 3 percent (from twenty-five to twenty-two). If you move from age forty-five to fifty-five, the change in percent is still 3 (from sixteen to thirteen), etc.

What all of that means is that, for males, the *amount of change* in volume, length, and circumference is *exactly* the same for *each and every year* of that graph. The only problem is that, in reality, the change is *not* perfectly uniform (exactly the same) each and every year. Ask any urologist or specialist in sexual dysfunctions.

Second, the type of graph presented, to be scientifically valid, would have had to have represented a longitudinal study. A longitudinal study is simply selecting a group and following that exact same group over a given period of time. A longitudinal study is opposed to a cross-sectional study, where a cross-section of the population is selected, measured only once at one point in time, and the results are tabulated. The longest, continuous-running, longitudinal study I know about is the Baltimore Longitudinal Study on Aging (BLSA), which has been in existence for approximately forty-five years. But look at the ages on this graph. They stretch from twenty to ninety, for a total of *seventy* years. The study by Drs. Bondil and Costa did not

YOUR PENIS IS SHRINKING!

It's a medical fact: The older you get, the less testosterone your body produces. And the less testosterone you have, the smaller your penis gets!

But now there's good news. Thanks to recent discoveries in nutritional science—such as supplementation with natural substances like zinc, cholestatin and orchic tissue, which stimulate the body's production of testosterone—it is now possible to stop and reverse the decline of testosterone levels.

This means new hope for men over 50 in the form of bigger erections and more youthful sexual function!

Penis Shrinkage Caused by Lower Testosterone Levels & Age

VOLUME 25%

LENGTH 19.8%

CIRCUMFERENCE 9%

AGE 20 30 40 50 60 70 80 90

In a landmark research study of 905 men conducted by Dr. P. Bondil and Dr. P. Costa of Harvard University and the Massachusetts Research Institute, it was shown how age-related decline in testosterone levels causes the penis to shrink dramatically as you grow older. However, this decline in penis size can now be corrected and potency can now be restored by taking advantage of an all-natural breakthrough that safely helps stimulate the production of testosterone.

7

run seventy years. If it did, it would mean that they were real whizzes and got out of medical school at age twenty-five, immediately began the study, and are both age ninety-five. They are not.

Further, to be a longitudinal study as implied, it would have meant that male subjects would have been selected for the study at age twenty, and then the three measurements (volume, length, and circumference) would had to have been taken annually on those *exact same men for the next seventy years*. That did not happen.

Since the flyer did not specify what type of study it was, the average reader is left to believe (hopefully) what the manufacturer wants you to believe; i.e., that the volume, length, and circumference decreases each and every year from age twenty to age ninety. That's simply not true. If you believe psychiatrists and psychologists, a significant amount of those three measurements have to do with what is above your neck, not below your waist.

Third, in my field of sports medicine, we know there are many things that can cause changes in those measurements. Examples would be smoking, diabetes, prescription drugs, alcohol, stress, lack of exercise; in fact, *any* condition that might result in a shrinking or blockage to the body's vascular system as well as what might affect its neurological system. The graph seems to imply that the mere process of aging is the sole cause of the decrease in the amounts, does it not? To put it to a point raised in the previous chapter, namely, "WORD:CURE," this ad fairly screams "OLDER: SMALLER."

And Gero Vita International is not the sole claimant to the "WORD:CURE" title. But some companies are a little more subtle. Herbal products have been added to the lines of One-A-Day (Bayer) and Centrum (Whitehall).

What Bayer does is simply put a few words on their box in big letters that state what your heath concern might be. The words are: Energy Formula; Menopause Health; Cholesterol Health; Prostate Health; Tension and Mood; Cold Season; Memory and Concentration; and Bone Strength. Each of those eight "titles" implies that: (a) if you've got this problem or concern (and here you would be self-diagnosing again), (b) buy our product and the problem or concern will go away. The "formulas" for each are a combination of vitamins, minerals, and herbs. It seems to make it oh-so-convenient to solve your problems just by taking these pills. In fact, what the ingredients may do is only support the entire body's systems in its attempt to attain and maintain the particular states addressed. Of course, there are absolutely no quantitative statements as to "how much" this support will be. And you won't see those statements because Bayer will not perform such a study because it would be too expensive and time-consuming (and the results of the study are not guaranteed in advance).

Whitehall uses a slightly different tactic in the visual presentation of its product line. What it does is emphasize the herb, such as ginseng, garlic, etc., and then follow it with a phrase that always begins "helps. . . ." As with Bayer, there are no statements as to "how much" (quantitatively) the help will be. Would you buy the product if a scientific study did, in fact, show a positive number that quantified the amount of help? Be careful. What if the number were 0.0005 percent? That number is a positive number; it fits the spirit and lettering of the ad, so the ad is not a lie or misleading. But the amount of the help is so small as to be, for all practical purposes, totally indiscernible. And, since you don't know the amount to begin with, why buy something that, right up front, can't tell you how much the change is going to be?

On a sidebar to the "WORD:CURE" concept, I have been disgusted for over twenty years at the advertising I see on TV during athletic events. During big football games, for example, you will see ads for some automotive manufacturer(s) and ads for beer manufacturers. I could condense all those ads into two words that would not be "WORD:CURE," but would describe the connection to a killer. Those two words are: "DRINKING:DRIVING."

*   *   *

There are killers in the herbal world that are being sold to you. Here's where the claims depart so far from reality as to put your life at risk. All too often, because of the unregulated status of the industry, the manufacturer and ad maker may not know the dangers of their product, but will not spend the money to find out. Let's make this a real tear-jerker. Let's assume the person pushing the product is doing so over the Internet and is, say, a disabled vet or a divorced mother with four young children. To you I say, "If you don't know the potential dangers of the product, don't push it." It's not going to be any value to my estate if I die from what you sold me, and you try and use as a defense that the independent rep who told you how to set up this neat MLM (Multi-Level Marketing) business and make tons of money told you the stuff was harmless. Let me put it succinctly, "Don't screw around with my life!"

Here are some examples of real killers.[2] Some kill you directly. Others do so indirectly, which occurs when you take some herbs that are touted as cures for deadly diseases. However, you totally disregard proven medical treatments, and the disease progresses to a point of no return, leaving you to die because you put your faith in an unproven remedy. As you read on, remember that these products have all been touted as being beneficial to us. That is the truth, if you can stand it. Yeah, tell it to the survivors.

Pennyroyal. Extracts of pennyroyal killed a college student at San Jose State University who took it to induce an abortion.[3]

Ephedrine. Used alone or with "harmless" substances like caffeine, ephedrine has killed countless people, who took it to lose weight as well as to "increase energy." Ephedrine is also called "Ephedra." It is used in products also known as ma huang, Chinese ephedra, and *Sida cordifolia.*

Siberian ginseng. This has caused birth defects when it was taken as an antidepressant and tranquilizer.

Kava. Large doses of this root extract have caused intoxication, nausea, muscle weakness, blurred vision, and drowsiness and has been implicated in a number of deaths.

Noni juice. This is actually the juice of the tropical plant *Morinda citrifolia*, and has been touted as a cure for cancer and a cancer inhibitor. People have died proving that one wrong.

Chaparral. This is a shrub and, when taken in tablet form, has been proven to cause hepatitis and may require a liver transplant for the consumer to stay alive.

Comfrey. It's like chaparral, does cause liver damage, and people have died from taking it.

Lobelia. It's also called Indian tobacco, and can lead to vomiting, convulsions, coma, and death.

(Herbal) "Fen-Phen." This stands for fenfluramine (brand name is Pondimin) and phentermine (brand name Redux). It has killed countless people. It is supposed to be off the market (at least products con-

taining it). The allure has been as a terrific weight-loss aid. If you want to try an interesting experiment, get on the Internet and type in "Redux," "Pondimin," or "Fen-Phen" and see if you can find anybody who is still selling it—even though all of it was supposed to be pulled from the market.

Stephania and magnolia. This is definitely toxic to the kidneys while being touted as a weight-loss product.

Yohimbe. This is promoted as an aphrodisiac (and one of the ingredients in the Testerex product I explained, above, from Gero Vita International). It's actually a plant that comes from West Africa. It can cause weakness, paralysis, gastrointestinal problems, and even psychosis.

Jin bu huan. It's promoted as a sedative, but has resulted in over-doses in children.

Shark cartilage. While not an herb, it has actually been advertised and (how dumb can some people be?) touted as a cancer preventive (by inhibiting the growth and development of blood vessels, which are needed to carry cancerous cells through the bloodstream). Bull. A book titled *Sharks Don't Get Cancer* received some exposure and even a sequel entitled *Sharks Still Don't Get Cancer.* Sharks *do* get cancer. Do I have to say anymore?

The list could go on and on, but the point I am making is this: without regulation, you are at risk. You are the last line of defense. Array your defenses wisely. To help you do that, you'll enjoy chapter 11, "Professional Advice: Who You Can Trust and Who You Can't Trust." You'll get some very valuable sources of information (some of the sources a virtual gold mine of information) on where to go to check something out before you take another step.

While not herbs per se, there are chemicals that are included with some herbs that can also kill you. *Do not, under any circumstances, buy, use, or give to anyone else* products known formally or "on the street" as Ecstasy (also known as "E" or "The Big E"), Serenity, Revitalize Plus, Thunder Nectar, SomatoPro, Weight Belt Cleaner, NRG3, GHRE, 5-HTP, or any product that contains GBL (gamma butyrolactone), BD (1,4 butanediol), or GHB (gamma hydroxybutyric). Manufacturers are creating and sometimes substituting life-threatening chemicals to "juice up" the rest of the product (or, sometimes, the foregoing are used as "stand-alone drugs"). The products and chemicals are pushed to give you a "party high" (whatever the hell that is), build muscle, lose weight, sedate you, calm you, brighten your outlook on life, etc. What they really do is cause excessive sweating, muscle cramps, irreversible brain damage, and death. They are being packaged with various herbs (and sometimes other supplements) supposedly to enhance the impact of the overall product. If you are seduced by the promise of the effect or the effect itself, your life is now a crapshoot every time you consume the product. On any supplement package—including herbs—*READ THE LABEL*. If any of the aforementioned killer substances is listed, *destroy that product*.

We all know what really fun people those Chinese Communists are. If the fact that differences in soil, growing, and harvesting do cause wide swings in potency of herbs grown anywhere in the world, you'll just love what the Chinese do with herbs (most Chinese medicines are herbal in nature).

In a fairly recent issue of the highly respected journal the *Lancet*, an article appears entitled: "Chinese Herbal Medicines Revisited: A Hong Kong Perspective."[4] What that article explains is the result of a collaborative effort by physicians at the Prince of Wales Hospital and the Chinese University of Hong Kong to review the published literature on the dangers of Chinese herbal and proprietary medicines. The results stated that these Chinese products were shipped around the world as well as being purchased on site by visitors to China. Ten of the 150 most commonly used toxic herbs are in that group. These products were also mixed in with traditional Western drugs (and no warnings were on the labels—even for toxic metals such as arsenic, mercury, lead, and cadmium). Further, even more toxic drugs than the ten of 150 were used because they were cheaper—yet *more* toxic. With the Chinese takeover of Hong Kong, you'd be nuts to buy anything they produced as "medicine" or herbs.

Should you see the word "standardized" (as in "standardized" amounts or "standardized" manufacturing quality control) on a label, it is essentially useless, except to push the product. Here's why: Because the supplement business is not regulated (as I've stated many times already), when the word "standardized" is used on a label for any supplements, it does not—repeat n-o-t—necessarily mean that the active ingredients of the herbs listed on the label are even present in *any* amount. What are present are what are known as "marker compounds" (some active ingredients) which may *not* be the herb's active ingredients. If that's the case, these marker compounds have absolutely nothing to do with the production of real benefits, if any at all, of the herb itself.

It is difficult to determine from the label what the active ingredients are, because some manufacturers have what they refer to as a "proprietary" standardization process which, they claim, means the active ingredients are actually present in each "pill." The process is proprietary in that it belongs solely to that manufacturer and is supposed to give the company a marketing edge over competitors who don't have that process. The problem is that the process is a secret outside the company, so there's no way to determine what the process is to determine if it works as advertised. Unfortunately, you the consumer are caught in the middle of a corporate security fight.

I don't want you to get too depressed. How about letting me liven things up a little bit with some ads, and I'll start with one of my favorites. I've seen this product advertised on TV as well as on the Internet. Unfortunately, the Internet ad has a prohibition against reproducing it, but I can give you the Internet address and let you see for yourself. The company is Reach4Life Enterprises and they market, among others, a product called "Grobust™." The Internet address is: http://reach4life.com/health.htm. When you get to the home page, look in the lower, far-right corner and you'll see the product name and where to click for more info.

What Grobust™ claims to do is increase the size of a woman's bust. The ingredients of Grobust™ are supposedly some herbs, whose relative strengths are never given. The truth of the matter is that estrogen—a hormone—can increase the size of a woman's breasts. Nothing else has been proven to do so. A friend of mine—a great Italian—when he saw the ad said, "Pizza."

I responded, "What?"

He replied, "Pizza will increase the size of a woman's breasts."

He seemed to be serious, so I cautiously asked him, "Are you telling me pizza will increase the size of a woman's breasts? You got any proof of that?"

He leaned back on the sofa and confidently said, "Sure. You seen my wife's (breasts) lately? It's all pizza, which has also increased the size of everything else she has. . . ."

As you scan the ad, look for the "grabber" words that you should now be familiar with, as well as other words and phrases used to entice you to buy. Do you see any results from any scientific studies to support the claims? Do you know anything about the institute that purports to support the claims? Do you know who heads that institute or his qualifications?

Let me quote from a personal correspondence from Stephen Barrett, M.D., who is a leading critic of fraud in healthcare. He is also board chairman of Quackwatch, Inc., which in my opinion has one of the top two sites on the Internet dealing with fraud in health care, found at: http://www.quackwatch.com.

In my query to Dr. Barrett regarding that institute and who heads it, he e-mailed me, on 16 May 1999, information regarding "Questionable Methods of Cancer Management" regarding "The Committee for Freedom of Choice in Medicine, Inc." I quote Dr. Barrett's communication to me, in part:

> Robert Bradford, the Committee's President, is also President of the Robert Bradford Research Institute (BRI). . . . Bradford is said to have received two honorary degrees: a "cultural doctorate in nutritional science" in 1983 from the World University and a "doctor of biochemistry degree" from Medicina Alternativa, an "international holistic medical group" in Sri Lanka. Although these degrees have no academic standing, the publications of both the Committee for Freedom of Choice in Medicine and the Bradford Institute identify him as "Dr. Bradford" or "Robert Bradford, DSc. . . ."
>
> The Bradford Research Institute . . . lists income of $13,819 in 1987, $17,518 in 1988, and $1,549 in 1989.

Do you, after reading their information, believe the claims or not?

* * *

The next ad is from an entity called Kid's Health Boutique,[5] whose headnote touts "Premium Nutrition for Kids." I pulled this ad off the Internet on 19 July 1999. It was found at address: http://209.130. 117.232/ websitep/kidsnutr.htm.

While I have reproduced it for you, because the colors used (light ones on dark background) make it somewhat difficult to read, I'll help you with it. The ad touts blue green algae, for kids, and for ADD (Attention Deficit Disorder).

How can the woman who supposedly runs the Kid's Health Boutique even advertise blue green algae for sale? The National Council Against Health Fraud has noted that they reviewed the literature on the toxic potential of that "herb." They did this because of continued complaints of weakness, diarrhea, numbness, tingling, and nausea in children who took blue green algae and products that contained it. What they found was that those reactions *were quite common*. The claims of blue green algae to cleanse and detoxify the body were absolutely false (I couldn't agree more). So, here we have someone pushing a product that has been *proven* to make kids sick. Like I said, it makes me sick, too. But you, dear reader, can ignore it before it claims your money and hurts your children.

Don't think I'm against all herbs and herbal products. I'm all for anything that has been scientifically proven to be safe and effective and under the umbrella of an honest ad. There are some herbs that are getting a lot of attention. For example, the herb St. John's Wort (*Hypericum perforatum*) has been found to be somewhat effective in mild cases of depression. There is no evidence that it is effective against severe depression. Danger has been shown where individuals take it while also taking prescription drugs such as Prozac and other antidepressants, and become more depressed.

Echinacea (ek-ih-NAY-see-uh), an herb in the daisy family, has shown some promise as being effective in combating the common cold when taken *orally*. The *injectable* echinacea does seem to increase certain cells in the immune system. In each situation, however, we are some distance from proving scientifically that it works for everybody, what the correct dosages should be, what the long-term effects of taking it are, and whether there are, as yet, any unknown harmful side effects.

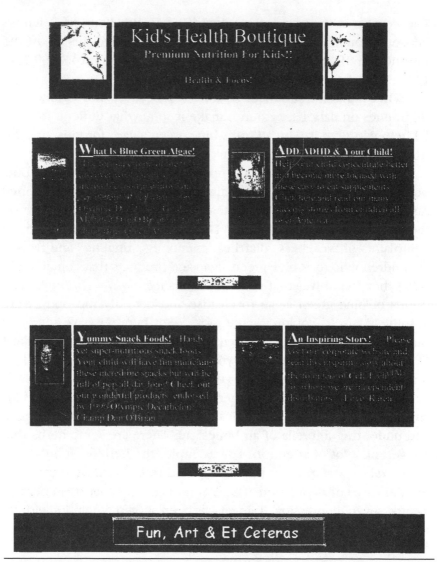

Ginseng shows some promise in mood elevation (elevating), reducing fasting blood glucose, and even reducing body weight. But, just as with echinacea, the same questions posed for it are yet to be answered for ginseng. The hucksters are not waiting. They are making the claims, couched in generalities, and you're acting as the human guinea pig—again.

Sometimes a reader doesn't believe what an author is trying to prove unless "outside experts" support what the author is saying. In addition to what Dr. Barrett e-mailed to me, let me quote from his excellent book *The Vitamin Pushers*. Dr. Barrett gives us a quote from Dr. Varro E. Tyler of Purdue University, who is a leading authority on plant medicines. Dr. Tyler is addressing the content of ads for herbal products:

> Practically all of these writings recommend large numbers of herbs for treatment based on hearsay, folklore, and tradition. The only criterion that seems to be avoided in these publications is scientific evidence. Some writings are so comprehensive and indiscriminate that they seem to recommend everything for anything. Even deadly poisonous herbs are sometimes touted as remedies, based on some outdated report or a misunderstanding of the facts. Particularly insidious is the myth that there is something almost magical about herbal drugs that prevents them, in their natural state, from harming people.
>
> *Many herbs contain hundreds or even thousands* [italics mine] of chemicals that have not been completely catalogued. Some of these chemicals may turn out to be useful as therapeutic agents, but others could well prove toxic. With safe and effective medicines available, treatment with herbs rarely makes sense. Moreover, many of the conditions for which herbs are recommended are not suitable for self-treatment. *Consumers are less likely to receive good value for money spent on herbal "remedies" than for almost any other health-related product* [italics mine].[6]

Dr. Tyler and I agree on three points; namely, that hucksters may *think* their products are safe, they may *want* them to be safe, but they don't *know* if they are safe.

Thus, in the name of money, they continue to push unproven products on you. And you continue to hope for the best while not knowing what the worst can be. You simply don't have an honest way to evaluate the risks if you don't know what they are. And that, dear reader, *is* the truth.

VIPS

The manufacturers of herbal supplements and remedies do not have to prove the safety or effectiveness of their products.

Some herbs have been proven to possess limited and mild beneficial effects on certain nonlife-threatening conditions, but some have been proven deadly when used in combination with other drugs and/or supplements.

No one knows for sure how many different herbs are on the market, singularly or in combination.

There is no database in any form (book, manual, computer database) that lists all known herbs and their real and potential interactions with prescription and nonprescription drugs.

There is absolutely no guarantee whatsoever as to the content, quality, purity, and absorption of an herb, either individually or in combination with any other supplement(s).

When looking at a graph or chart, analyze it and see if it refers to any accompanying text, and see whether the results are even feasible, if not absolutely incorrect.

The "WORD:CURE" connection is one of the main ways you get duped.

Some herbs have been proven to be killers. No question about it.

It bears repeating! Do not, under any circumstances, buy, use, or give to anyone else products known formally or "on the street" as Ecstasy (also known as "E" or "The Big E"), Serenity, Revitalize Plus, Thunder Nectar, SomatoPro, Weight Belt Cleaner, NRG3, GHRE, 5-HTP, or any product that contains GBL (gamma butyrolactone), BD (1,4 butanediol), or GHB (gamma hydroxybutyric). On any supplement package—including herbs—*READ THE LABEL*. If any of the aforementioned killer substances is listed, *destroy that product.*

Stay away from herbs or herbal medicines from the People's Republic of China.

The word "standardized" on a label is your assurance of nothing.

Many herbs contain hundreds or even thousands of chemicals that have not been completely catalogued.

Consumers are less likely to receive good value for money spent on herbal "remedies" than for almost any other health-related product.

You don't have any honest way to evaluate the risks of any herb if you don't know what they are.

As you read through the next chapter, be aware that dollars are at stake—your dollars. Whereas you might spend only a few bucks on a onetime purchase of a bottle of supplements, exercise equipment can easily run into the hundreds of dollars for a single purchase.

The impact on your body is different with supplements vis-à-vis exercise equipment. The former is primarily involved in biochemistry. The latter is primarily involved in physiology (function) and biomechanics (how it works). Thus, the focus of the ads is different, but the aim of the manufacturer is the same—to separate you from your money with promises.

NOTES

1. Gero Vita International ad for Testerex. Ad taken from brochure received by the author in September 1999.

2. Sources of this information include: Arnot Ogden Medical Center (www.aomc.org/NewsRelease/HerbalFen-Phen.html), FDA, Mayo Clinic (www.mayohealth.org/mayo/9703/htm/herb_sb.htm), National Council Against Health Fraud (NCAHF) (http://ncahf.org/nl/nlindex.html), and Quackwatch.com.

3. *San Jose Mercury News*, 20 August 1994.

4. "Chinese Herbal Medicines Revisited: A Hong Kong Perspective," *Lancet* 3452 (1993): 1532–34.

5. Kid's Health Boutique ad for blue green algae products (and others). Internet advertisement printed from address: http://209.130.117.232/websitep/kidsnutr.htm [19 July 1999], p. 1 of 2.

6. Stephen Barrett and Victor Herbert, *The Vitamin Pushers: How the "Health Food" Industry Is Selling America a Bill of Goods* (Amherst, N.Y.: Prometheus Books, 1994), p. 163.

8   FITNESS EQUIPMENT
Helpful, Harmful, or Hype?

F ID, ROM, and IR. These are not acronyms dealing with computers, but the necessary elements in any exercise program (and the equipment used) to achieve your greatest benefits from the piece of equipment that is being advertised. If you keep this in mind, you'll quickly learn that some advertised equipment—regardless of the claims—must necessarily fall short of these claims.

In FID, "F" stands for "frequency"; "I" stands for "intensity"; "D" stands for "duration." The frequency refers to how often you exercise in a given time period, such as once a week, twice a week, four times a month, etc. The intensity refers to "how hard" you exercise. Duration refers to the amount of time you exercise without stopping, such as five seconds, one minute, fifteen minutes, etc. Here's an example. Assume you are lifting weights. You work out three times a week. That is your frequency. Assume you only do one exercise, say, the bench press. You do three sets of ten repetitions with 150 pounds on the bar. That is your intensity. Last, assume that this workout takes you five minutes to complete the three sets of ten repetitions. That is your duration.

Here's another quick example. Assume you exercise by walking three times a week (frequency). You walk at the pace of three miles per hour (intensity). You walk continuously for thirty minutes (duration).

It's extremely important to understand that each of the three terms—frequency, intensity, and duration—are interrelated. In fact, they are also interdependent.

ROM stands for Range of Motion. This is the distance that a particular part of your body can move through a given exercise. For example, if you are doing sit-ups and you begin by lying on your back on the floor with your legs extended straight (knees not bent), your ROM would be (forward) as far as you can bring your upper body up and then forward toward your feet. The rearward motion would go only as far as the floor, which, of course, stops the body from moving any further. Your ROM may be, as in this case, limited by your degree of flexibility. If you can only curl your body fifteen degrees off the floor, that's it. That's as far as you go. Your ROM is only fifteen degrees from the starting point. If you're quite flexible, you might be able to curl your body so far forward as to be able to touch your forehead to the front of your legs (I hate people who can do that). If you are one of these people, your ROM is about 180 degrees.

IR stands for Increasing Resistance. For example, if you're lifting weights and you bench press 100 pounds, then add 10 pounds of plates, you have increased the resistance by 10 pounds.

If you have ever done any exercising, or even just read a lot about it, the foregoing may seem painfully simple, if not outright dull. Beware. An understanding of these elements is absolutely necessary to spot a phony ad. The hucksters know this. This is why you will seldom see FID, ROM, or IR mentioned in any of the ads. There are other elements, such as "sticking point," which I will cover later in this chapter, which may or may not exist relative to any given exercise. The hucksters get rich simply by ignoring fact and including only what they think will work as selling points.

"Pssst. Hey, Sucker. Yeah, you. C'mere. How'd ya like to have rock-hard abs in only three minutes a day? It's fast. It's easy. In no time at all, your fat will just melt away. This amazing, incredible, fantastic, revolutionary abdominal machine can give you the abs you've always wanted. Just think what you'll feel like when you have abs like Big Mike, here. And you also get this complete, four-second video showing you how much fun you'll have losing those inches. And, for the first hundred callers, we'll throw in—absolutely free—our unbelievable, technologically advanced tape measure *plus* this sturdy, hand-painted, 100 percent real cotton towel to wipe the sweat out of your eyes, just for calling. This is a $6,000 value, all for just three easy payments of $29.95. DO IT NOW! YOU CAN'T AFFORD TO MISS THIS FANTASTIC OFFER!"

Did you get duped by one of those stupid ads? Don't feel bad. Millions of people spent money on the ab rollers, ab crunchers, ab (whatever), and got . . . disappointed (not to mention duped). I've seen several surveys that showed the waist is the most often cited part of the anatomy people want to change (make smaller, harder, slimmer, etc.). The hucksters jumped all over that one. The public apparently pays a lot of attention to its own stomach ("abs" for "abdominals"), but doesn't understand its anatomy, physiology, or biomechanics. In point of fact, all of these claims about ab machines are doomed to failure before they are ever shouted.

Here's why: The abdominal area is a composite of four paired sets of muscles. And each paired set has muscle fibers that run in a different direction. Imagine that you are standing upright and looking at yourself in a full-length mirror. Look at the image in the mirror and look at your "stomach area." If I peeled away the outer layers of skin and fat in that stomach area in the image in the mirror, here's what that image would look like. You'd first see the outermost set of abdominal muscles called the *external obliques*. (Remember, you are seeing what is in the mirror.) The set of external obliques on the right side has muscle fibers that run from your side, downward to the left at about a forty-five-degree angle, toward the centerline of your body. The set on the other side runs from your side, downward to the right, toward the center of your body. Underneath the external obliques lie the *internal obliques*, and their muscle fibers on each side of your body run in exactly the *opposite* direction as the external obliques, also at a forty-five-degree (downward) angle. If you could see both the external and internal obliques at the same time, their muscle fibers would form an "X" on each side of your body—the external obliques being on top.

Underneath the internal obliques lie the *tranversus abdominis*. Their muscle fibers do not run downward to the left or right, but are actually *parallel*; i.e., they run left to right *across* the abdominal area, not angled downward like the obliques.

Last, the *rectus abdominis* lie underneath the transversus abdominis and, you guessed it, they run up and down (at right angles to the transverse abdominis).

So, if you saw all four sets of muscles on just one side, it would look like an "X" lying on top of a big "+" sign.

Can't these nifty abdominal machines work all those muscles? Yep, but not much. They fail *miserably* as to intensity, ROM, and increasing resistance. We actually measured some of those machines ("machines" seems too complicated a word for something that is just some pipe and padding with essentially no moving parts). We found that, when a person tried to do the sit-up or "crunch" (whether lifting their upper body straight or in a twist position), they could barely raise their upper body off the floor more than thirty degrees. Therefore, the ROM was only one-sixth the full ROM of a full sit-up. Because the ROM was severely limited, so too was the intensity. Except for one machine, there was no way to increase the resistance. To work the abdominal muscles harder, you could *only* do more repetitions, which simply made the workout time that much longer. So much for the ". . . three minutes a day . . ." or whatever time was in the ad. Since work is determined by the amount of force it takes to move a mass over a distance, the force could never increase because the mass (the weight of your upper body) is essentially unchanged, and the distance (ROM) remains the same.

If that weren't bad enough, the machines have a pad on which to rest your neck. This means that, as you begin the exercise movement, the uppermost part of your body is already bending in toward your chest. What this does, speaking biomechanically, is to prevent you from doing a full ROM. The ads tout that it keeps your neck steady. Big deal. So does clasping your hands behind your head and holding your neck steady (as when you do regular sit-ups).

The hucksters touted how safe it was to use their machines for people with weak backs and backs that hurt. Want to know the most common complaint by patients to their physicians? It's back pain. Know what causes most back pain? It's weak abdominal muscles. So now we have this machine that limits the intensity, ROM, and IR. What does that do? *It severely limits the strengthening of the abdominal and the back muscles—just the opposite of what the hucksters are touting.* Have you heard any people on ads touting how their machine works the muscles of the mid- and lower *back—* especially the *latissimus dorsi* and the lower-down *erector spinae?* You won't, and the reason you won't is that those back muscles hardly move when you are working on those abs machines.

If your physician says you have a weak back, but are able to do limited ROM sit-ups (we call them "crunches"—limited in ROM with more tucking of the chin toward the chest), you need to strengthen the back *and* abdominal muscles and you do that by exercising those muscles through 180 degrees of motion (if you can go that far), not thirty degrees.

Though this is not scientific, have you seen anybody in the last three years (the time these machines have been on the market) who has gotten "rock-hard abs," "abs that look like the models in the ads," or had the fat just "melt away," just from using that machine? I haven't, nor do I expect to.

World-class bodybuilders spend approximately four hours per day working out. If these ab machines were so great, why haven't they forsaken regular sit-ups, decline sit-ups, Roman Chairs, and the like for their abs? It would only make sense to trade hours per week working your abs if you could get the same result in only minutes with those whiz-bang, nifty, super-duper, it's-so-easy abdominal machines.

To put it bluntly, don't waste your money on those machines. You can do everything—and more—without the machine than you can with it. The machines restrict your motion and options and limit your progress. Save your money and a lot of frustration.

A few more points to keep you from getting duped: Genetics determines where your fat cells are located and how many you have. Unfortunately, some people have a lot of fat cells between their stomach's outer skin and the various sets of abdominal muscles. What this does is—to a great degree—limit how small that person can make their waist and whether the abdominal muscles underneath will ever "show through." I have known patients who literally did thousands of sit-ups a month and never had that "washboard" stomach. *Be careful.* What I just said is only partially true. Those people *did* have washboard stomachs, you just couldn't see the muscles underneath the fat.

I just used another tactic that is terribly effective in getting you to spend your money. What happens is this: The ads will just be cruising along blabbing away at how neat their machine is, many times employing some supposed expert or celebrity. You trust them (why, I don't know), so you are not paying very close attention. You're not analyzing as they speak. All of a sudden they slip something in and hope it goes right by you. It might be in the form of a disclaimer, so they have done their legal duty by giving the disclaimer. You will not see this disclaimer (or extremely quick statement that the machine only works some of the time on some people), results can and will vary; the person used as the model got results that were anything but the usual, expected results by the majority of users.

You will never hear any huckster explain that. They want you to believe that they have the answer to your problem. The one machine that will do exactly what you want it to do—fast, without pain, seemingly without effort. They are lying to you.

What follows is what I consider to be the greatest misrepresentation (or outright lie) in the entire industry.

Here it is: ". . . this (name of piece of equipment) will add muscle. . . ." If you didn't notice the problem with that phrase, go back and read it s-l-o-w-l-y. Ladies and gentlemen, *no piece of exercise equipment in the entire history of the world has ever added a single muscle to anybody. Not once. Not ever.*

Don't go easy on the manufacturer and/or ad maker. They are the ones who have all the time and resources to make the ad, which includes research, writing, and editing.

The scientific fact is simply that you are born with all the muscles you're ever going to have. No piece of equipment can add muscle to your body. Keep in mind that when advertisers speak of adding muscle, they are referring to adding bulk, not more individual muscles, but that's not the idea you might perceive. Taking this a step further, the hucksters will also hit you with the second greatest misrepresentation (or outright lie) in the entire industry: ". . . this (name of piece of equipment) will build muscle. . . ." *No it will not build anything. Protein, made from amino acids, builds muscle. Period.* In fact, exercise itself—especially strenuous resistance exercise (like heavy weightlifting)—absolutely tears down your muscles. That is why we experts keep telling people to allow at least one day of rest between strenuous bouts of exercise and e-a-t g-o-o-d f-o-o-d. That food will provide the absolutely necessary substances to allow your body to recover after those tough exercise sessions.

Here is what exercise machines do (and I'll include free weights here), and it is all they do. They may increase the size of your muscle. And the amount of increase in size is dependent on three sets of information which affect the potential growth of your muscles: genetics, diet, and the FID/ROM/IR.

There is nothing magical about any of the information on the preceding pages. The only magical trick is how people take basic, simple, irrefutable truth and twist it, ignore it, deemphasize it, and make a lot of money from ignorant people.

The hucksters who manufacture and sell "self-contained gyms" or "complete or total workout (whatever)" have a field day messing with your mind. The reason they get away with it is that their piece of equipment is presented on several premises. Those premises are:

- That the equipment is terribly convenient because they are an "all-in-one" piece of equipment;
- That the piece of equipment gives you a virtually unlimited number of possible ways to exercise your various muscle groups; thus, it is the most versatile piece of equipment ever built;
- You are far safer than using those dirty, nasty, clangy, rusty, old free weights;
- That the equipment is so technologically advanced that you'll never need to buy another piece of exercise equipment for as long as you live;
- You'll be able to make startling improvement and progress toward your goal of (fill in the blank) weight loss, aerobic conditioning, flexibility, muscular definition, "spot reducing," and almost anything else they can dream up for you.

Every one of these premises is absolutely false.

To prove it let's take a look at a "complete" piece of exercise equipment called the Total Gym 2000®, manufactured by Total Fitness

Gyms, Inc. I saw the ad on 30 August 1999, on Times-Warner Cable channel 38, in the Atlanta viewing area, from approximately 8 A.M. to 8:30 A.M. Yes, the ad was almost one-half hour in length. Not only did viewers get to see the equipment in use, they were even "treated" to watching model Christie Brinkley and actor Chuck Norris expounding its virtues and working out on the machine (all for a price—they got paid to do the ad, as a graphic during the ad did show). The machine basically consists of a board you sit/lie on, and, using pulleys, inclining the board (which slides), and your own body weight, you move your body (or parts thereof) back and forth. Big deal.

Ms. Brinkley positively gushed all the right phrases: ". . . (working out on the machine) makes your workouts faster and easier than you've ever imagined possible," "You'll look and feel better than you ever thought possible," and "It's not boring or exhausting." You can see how improbable those statements are. In fact, as to the last statement, she later stated that she had worked her muscles ". . . to exhaustion." Well, which is it, Christie, exhausting or not?

She later made a major faux pas when she mentioned that she had recently given birth and that she ". . . only had eight more pounds to lose and I'm going to lose it all with nothing but the Total Gym 2000®." She's either lying, is ignorant, or doesn't plan on losing that weight for over *two years*. Read that sentence again. *Dr. Forness, did you really mean to say that it would take her over two years to lose eight pounds if she only used the machine?*

That's exactly what I said, and I'm going to prove it.

During that ad, it was stated that, if you purchased the Total Gym 2000®, you would also get a free (uh-huh) video describing the six-to eight-minute workout you should follow. There was another man in the ad. Everybody was simply "amazed" at how fast, easy, and effective the machine is. How can you tell how fast, easy, and effective something is by just standing around and watching somebody else work out on a piece of equipment? Just remember that the next time some huckster claims to be able to provide you with such a piece of equipment.

I'm going to be generous and say that Ms. Brinkley is going to work out the longer period—eight minutes—and not the shorter time period of six minutes. Further, I am going to say she works out every single day. I don't know her exact weight (she never said), but I'll assume it's 130 pounds, so she wants to get down to 122 pounds.

The good people at the American College of Sports Medicine provide many texts on exercise and its effects. From various texts, I present you with the proof of how long it will take to lose eight pounds, given Ms. Brinkley's situation.

One pound equals 3,500 calories, so she needs to expend 28,000 calories (8 times 3,500).

The formula for determining calories expended in one minute is:

$$\text{kcal/min} = VO_2(\text{in liters per minute}) \times 5 \text{ kcal per liter}$$

VO_2 stands for "oxygen uptake" which measures energy expended. It is the standard, accepted measure in the (legitimate) health and fitness industry.

To find VO_2, you find the metabolic effort and multiply it by the constant number, 3.5. The metabolic effort is called a "MET" (not the baseball player) and stands for "metabolic equivalent." One MET is the amount of energy your body expends when you are totally at rest. Anything else you do is a multiple of that 1 MET. For example, working out lightly with resistance equipment (and she, Chuck Norris, and the other guy kept saying how "easy" and "effortless" it was—their words, not mine) is equivalent to 4.0 METs. So, 4.0×3.5 gives us a VO_2 of 14.0.

To convert that VO_2 into liters per minute, use the formula:

$$VO_2(\text{in liters per min}) = VO_2 \times (\text{body weight in kilograms}/1000)$$

Her body weight is 130 pounds. To get kilograms, divide the body weight by 2.2, and you get 59.09 kilograms. Now, put the VO_2 (14.0) and the body weight in kilograms (59.09) into the formula above, and you get:

$$VO_2(\text{in liters per min}) = 14.0 \times (59.09 /1000)$$

$$VO_2(\text{in liters per min}) = 14.0 \times (0.059)$$

$$VO_2(\text{in liters per min}) = 0.826$$

Now put the 0.826 into the formula with which I began this proof and you get:

$$kcal/min = VO_2(\text{in liters per minute}) \times 5 \text{ kcal per liter}$$

$$kcal/min = 0.826 \times 5 \text{ kcal per liter}$$

$$kcal/min = 4.13$$

Okay, sports fans, Ms. Brinkley will expend 4.13 calories per minute for every minute she works out on the Total Gym 2000®. Since she needs to expend 28,000 calories, simply divide 28,000 by 4.13 kcal/min, and you get 6,779.66 minutes. That's how many minutes she has to work out to lose the eight pounds (28,000 calories). Remember, *she* was the one who said she was going to lose that weight doing *nothing but* working out on the Total Gym 2000®.

Folks, do one more computation with me. Since she's going to work out eight minutes per day, divide 6,779.66 by 8 and you get (drumroll please) *847.46. That's the number of days it will take her to lose the eight pounds. That's over twenty-eight months, and that is over two years.*

You can use these formulas for yourself. To help you, remember that in chapter 3 I told you about the American College of Sports Medicine's *Resource Manual for Guidelines for Exercise Testing and Prescription*, where all the METs are listed.

Now I ask you, would you buy that machine, or any machine, which would only provide such long, slow progress?

The ad also claimed that the six-to-eight-minute workout per day on the Total Gym 2000® was equivalent to a twenty-minute aerobic workout. That's pure baloney. I could use the same formulas from the previous pages and prove it. I'm telling you, folks, hucksters will say anything they can get away with unless somebody calls them on it. I just did.

If that weren't enough, this "versatile" machine requires the users to use their own body weight as the resistance for the workout. What if you want to increase the resistance? Ah, the machine has a series of "incline settings" to make the effort harder. Don't hurt yourself. And you *could* hurt yourself because those angles of incline start at 4 percent and increase up to 60 percent, but the increase is not continuous. You have only seven settings in that total range. That means each setting is an increase in incline level of 8 percent (60 minus 4, divided by 7). If you weigh 150 pounds, that means each higher incline setting increases the resistance by 8 percent (or twelve pounds). In many exercises that a person would do with dumbbells (bicep curls, butterflies, chest pullovers, etc.), you should *never* increase the resistance by more than 5 percent when going from one set of an exercise to the next. If you do, you stand a real good chance of tearing your connective tissue (ligaments, cartilage, and tendons).

If you go back to FID, ROM, and IR, how many of these necessary elements are lacking or diluted with that machine, based on what I've told you? You should have found that all but two—frequency and duration—are lacking or diluted.

All right, I've just given you some more ways you can be (or already have been) duped. Be aware that any machine that touts results as being "fast" and "easy" is not, because anything that violates or dilutes the basic tenets of FID, ROM, and IR is just not very effective. You can't have fast and easy and quick results. They are absolutely contradictory to the anatomy, physiology, and biomechanics of the human body.

Here are more things to watch out for, and they can hurt you. Earlier in this chapter I mentioned "sticking points." A sticking point is the location in any exercise where the movement against the resistance is most difficult. For example, if you want to do a bench press, the sticking point is when the bar is resting on your chest. In the bicep curl, it is where your arm(s) are fully extended with no bend in your elbow. In the sit-up, it's where you first try to bend your upper body toward your lower body (like when you are lying on the floor and just begin to lift your upper body off the floor). In the "squat" (deep knee bends with weight on your shoulders) it is where your knees are bent as far as they can go. Please pay attention to this: *You never, ever, ever want to begin any resistance exercise where your body is at the sticking point.*

Where you can get duped again—and possibly tear your connective tissue—is when you get suckered into buying any piece of resistance exercise equipment where you begin an exercise at the sticking point. A product called Bowflex® is a perfect example (as is the Total Gym 2000®). I saw an ad for Bowflex® on 24 May 1999 on Time-Warner cable channel 31, in the Atlanta area, between 10 A.M. and 10:15 A.M. When you try and do the bench-press exercise, you absolutely *start* in the sticking-point position. In fact, the two handles you grip (one with each hand) are positioned so you actually are trying to start the movement with your hands farther *behind* your chest than you could with a bar that your hands would grip. That puts the greatest strain on your muscles and connective tissue at the sticking point (also consider it the point where you have the greatest amount of inertia to overcome).

The ad content for Bowflex® almost defied belief. Here's an incredible quote from the ad: "You need to add muscle to lose fat." Isn't that beyond belief? I made the case, above, that no piece of exercise equipment has ever, or will ever, *add* any muscle to any human body. And the other point is that there is absolutely no cause-effect between adding muscle and losing fat. Even if they had correctly said, ". . . *developing* muscle . . ." that changes nothing. It is so easy to prove that you can lose (really meaning "reduce") fat without developing any muscle. In point of scientific fact, if you want to lose fat quickly, you can do so while *at the same time* reducing the size of your muscles. Your body doesn't work any other way when you lose weight, part in fat, part in muscle.

Other ridiculous claims made during the Bowflex® ad—all designed to dupe the unsuspecting, innocent, ignorant viewing audience—were: "Nothing can be easier"; "It only takes twenty minutes a day"; "Completely reshape your body." Uh-huh.

Look at the ad for Soloflex®.[1] The female is at the sticking point for a behind-the-neck press. That exercise should begin with the arms fully extended over her head. It's just the opposite. Most of the exercises with the Soloflex® require you to *begin* at the sticking point. I wouldn't use a Bowflex®, a Soloflex®, a Total Gym 2000®, or any other exercise machine, regardless of the manufacturer, even if I got it free.

Let me put it succinctly: In forty years of being exposed to, analyzing, and using many of the different types of resistance exercise equipment, there is *nothing* that has been able to beat free weights, which are always a lot cheaper than the other types of "equipment." Most of the nonfree-weight equipment is hype. Pure and simple. Free weights allow greater range of motion, greater variability in grips of lifting bars, and greater variability in increase and decrease of resistance between sets; free weights are cheaper and there is nothing to wear out; free weights also allow the lifter to "cheat" on heavy lifts—which is creating momentum to help overcome the inertia of the heavy weight.

All the pulleys, bands (made of some form of elastic substance), pads, handles, boards, tubes, cams, and other accessories to the equipment is not as effective—when put to the test of FID *and* ROM *and* IR—as free weights. That, too, is pure and simple.

Think for a moment of a word—*fitness*—and see what, if any, definition that word conjures up in your mind. That word is bantered all over the ballpark. I doubt if many people, including the hucksters, even know what the word means. I give you the meaning: Fitness refers to one muscle, and only one muscle—your heart. The stronger that muscle, the more fit you are. The *only* way you can make any muscle in your body stronger is by exercising that muscle against a heavier and heavier (increasing) resistance.

Here's why. This is what happens when you exercise: When you want to make your skeletal muscles stronger, you must either lift heavier weights or press those muscles against resistance in weight machines. The only way to strengthen your heart muscle is to exercise it. As you begin exercising, the skeletal muscles squeeze the blood from the veins that are near them and push that blood to your heart. The heart muscle has to squeeze faster and harder to pump that increase in blood supply through the rest of your body. So, the harder you exercise, the faster and harder your heart beats (squeezes and relaxes, squeezes and relaxes). This continues for as long as you continue exercising. Therefore, fitness is determined more by how hard you exercise than by how long you exercise. You might walk slowly for thirty minutes and not improve your fitness anywhere near what pressing 150 pounds for only five minutes would do (and most of us could never press any fairly heavy weight for five minutes continuously).

If any ad talks about making you "fit" or "more fit" or "increase your

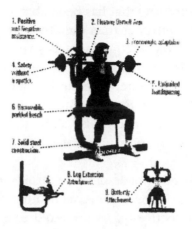

1. Positive and Negative resistance. Soloflex Weightstraps give you full positive and negative resistance. Both forms of resistance have been shown by science to be necessary for maximum muscle growth. You get positive resistance on the power stroke, and negative resistance on the return stroke. And, in independent studies, Soloflex Weightstraps have been shown to provide the same muscle gains as freeweight iron plates.

2. Floating Barbell Arm. Our patented floating barbell arm, like a freeweight barbell, requires you to supply the balance in weightlifting. It won't let your stronger side cheat for your weak side, insuring symmetrical body development.

3. Freeweight adaptable. Many owners like using the Soloflex Muscle Machine with freeweight plates, which slide easily on the machine. Your Soloflex comes standard with two iron plate attachment rods. These let you lift on your Soloflex with iron plates alone, or with a combination of plates and weightstraps.

4. Safety without a spotter. The Soloflex Muscle Machine introduced safe, home weightlifting to Americans back in 1978. The machine's patented design lets you lift as much weight as you like, without a spotter. You're secure in the knowledge that bar can't fall on you in during such important exercises as the bench press and squats.

5. Unlimited handspacing. The straight Soloflex Barbell Arm, like a freeweight barbell, lets you move your hands anywhere you like. This unlimited handspacing is required to get the full benefit out of many weightlifting exercises.

6. Removable padded bench. The comfortable Soloflex bench goes on and off quickly and easily, to let you do dozens of exercises. You can incline the bench for bench presses and crunches. Or, take the bench off to accommodate standing bicep curls, squats, calf raises, pull ups, and many other important weightlifting favorites.

7. Solid steel construction. Soloflex's superior construction is unrivaled by any competitor. The Soloflex Muscle Machine, like all Soloflex products, is backed by a 5-year warranty.

fitness," don't get suckered. To get or become more fit, you've got to work out harder and harder. In fact, if you really do a good hard workout, that workout actually *damages* your muscles, and it takes the average person approximately forty-eight hours to recover. I'm not kidding. Fibers in the muscles actually suffer minute tears, which repair themselves in one to two days, on average. Muscles develop—become larger—with movement against heavier and heavier resistance, and become smaller and weaker with disuse, over time. Hard, vigorous exercise does damage your muscles, but the damage should never be permanent. No huckster will ever tell you his machine damages your muscles. That may be true, especially if the exercises are truly so easy as to not force your muscles to develop. And that, ladies and gentlemen, has just blown the phony ads right out of the water.

Treadmills have enjoyed some justifiable success, though they are certainly not inexpensive, with some models costing several thousand dollars. In response to the cost factor, the industry has come out with what are called "elliptical trainers," machines that allow the user to stride at any speed, with motion of the lower legs and feet describing an ellipse; hence the name "elliptical" trainer. An ellipse is a somewhat round shape, but not a circle; much more like a football as viewed from its side. There are really five types of machines—cross-country skiing machines, elliptical trainers, treadmills, stairsteppers, and cycle ergometers (essentially stationary bicycles)—that compete with each other as cardiovascular equipment. In research studies, the treadmill and the elliptical trainers produced almost the same rates of oxygen consumption, caloric expenditure, and heart rate, superior to the stairstepper and the cycle ergometer. A great article—"Elliptical Trainers: Giving the Treadmill a Run for Its Money," by Vicki Pierson—can be found at http://primusweb.com/fitnesspartner/library/equipment/elliptical.htm.

The elliptical trainer is clearly superior to the treadmill in having less than half the impact forces encountered by the lower legs. This may be crucial with people who have arthritis, joint pain, swelling, or other types of orthopedic injury. With an elliptical trainer, both feet are *always* in contact with the surfaces of the machine on which they are placed—unlike a treadmill where the feet leave the running surface, just as feet do in running over the ground.

What Pierson's article does not show, and the manufacturers do not admit, is that there is a critical shortcoming with the elliptical trainers as compared with the treadmills. With the elliptical trainers, the length of your stride is fixed; i.e., your ROM is constant. You can't lengthen your stride if you want to "run" faster. Early in my training, I learned that running speed is the product of stride length and stride frequency. When you try running at a rate of more than a six-minute mile (which is a fairly good clip), you must lengthen your stride over that at slower speeds. I also learned that people will suffer leg pains when they cycle or use an elliptical trainer at a given speed, then try and run at that same speed. This is so because, as your stride lengthens, your ROM increases, stretching muscles further than they ever were on the bike or elliptical trainer, causing soreness.

Too many people were having problems with balance with the cross-country skiing machines, and their sales have really fallen off with the advent of elliptical trainers.

Where you don't want to get duped is when hucksters tout building upper body strength and flexibility. Because there is no IR (increasing resistance) relative to the upper body and no stride-length increase possible (except with the treadmill), the range of motion is fixed.

It's unfortunate that machines like the elliptical trainers have a lot of good points, but these good points are emphasized at the expense of the misrepresentations. One ad for an elliptical trainer touted the ". . . forward and reverse, upper body, constant rotation, cyclical aerobic enhancer. . . ." Oh, for pete's sake, all that means is that you have a pair of bars your hands rest on that move back and forth.

One of the most incredible ads for stretching believability past the breaking point comes to us from the inventor of the HoloBarre System™. Look at the ad below.[2] Does the fact that this HoloBarre™ is nothing but a bar you mount in a doorway tell you anything? If you want to read the many, many pages of the ad and the links connected to it, just get on the Internet at address: http://www.holobarre.com and go at it. I truly think this is one of the sillier products I've ever seen in my entire career.

When I read through the entire text of the ad for this "equipment," several times I found myself wondering whether or not it was for real. I pictured a couple of guys in a bar on a slow night and one saying to the other, "Hey Ernie. Why don't we take a piece of straight pipe, make up a jazzy ad for it, stick it on the Internet, and see how many suckers will take the bait?"

If you wonder how I can waste valuable time analyzing these stupid ads, just say that's "it's a lousy job, but somebody's gotta do it." Actually, some of the ads are funnier than the junk that is fobbed off as comedy on TV. Look at the first page I printed. First of all, how did the guy hanging upside down on the bar get up there? More importantly, how does he get down? Next, look at the beginning of the last paragraph on that page. It is not possible that a stationary bar can "facilitate virtually *every exercise imaginable*." When I did some wrestling, we had to do "neck bridges." Neck bridges are neck-strengthening exercises where you lie flat on the floor, on your back, and you raise your entire body off the floor using only the soles of your feet and your neck—so your feet and the back of your head are the only parts of your body in contact with the floor. No way can you do it on that bar. When I was playing football, we had "reach-out drills." A reach-out drill is performed standing, feet spread apart, and both hands (palms out) are violently thrust forward (as if to ward off a blocker) and then the hands and arms throw off the blocker from contact with you. No way can you do those on/with that bar.

Now look at the top of the second page. "HoloBarre can do 99% of the exercises that 99 percent of the population needs." I tried, dear readers. I really tried to think of what those exercises were that the 99 percent consisted of, as well as whomever determined exactly what exercises the population needs. I admit I couldn't create such a list.

You can also get duped in such a subtle way that, even watching someone working out on one of the "all-in-one" pieces of exercise equipment, you don't know *how* you're being duped. It has everything to do with range of motion, intensity, and a geometric form.

Assume I'm standing upright, with my arms extended straight down at my sides. I put a flashlight in my right hand. You are standing at my right side, maybe six feet away, facing me from the side. I turn my right hand so the head of the flashlight is pointing at you. Now, let's turn out the lights. If I do a movement such as a

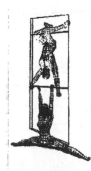

You will learn

1. how your body (and exercise equipment) works mechanically, as well as a wide range of fitness, nutrition, and CONSUMER issues;
2. interesting physical principles with far-reaching consequences;
3. important points of philosophy and perspective on health and fitness;
4. about the health & fitness industry in general.
Oh! And I almost forgot....
5. how to become stronger and healthier than with any other system, and without gadgets......

The HoloBarre System is an amalgamation of these principles, so much so that understanding your body virtually implies knowing the full capabilities of the HoloBarre, and, vice-versa.

In a doorway and without clutter or gadgets, The HoloBarre System enables a panoramic array of exercises, stretches, and physical therapy, rehab, and chiropractic methods. The Olympic athlete, the harried business person, the octogenarian, and the wheelchair bound are all equally embraced by this system.

Not only does the HoloBarre facilitate virtually **every exercise imaginable**, it allows a given exercise to be performed in numerous, even dozens of different ways, with uncountable variations! It is the only system that allows you to be **physically creative** with ordinary and *extraordinary* exercise!

and we LOVE e-mail, and answer all mail!

What's new on this site?

The Big Picture tells you why the HoloBarre exists, and gives you a thumbnail sketch about what, in part, motivates us, and hopefully what will help motivate you.

The Overview describes how and why the HoloBarre works, along with an example of the inventor's own super-efficient exercise routine.

The Description, specs, and installation

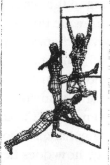

The Free Instructional Video will leave you astonished at how much you can do with so little equipment!

The Only *Infinitely Versatile* Exercise System, Facilitating Virtually Every Exercise, Stretch, and Position in Existence....all in a Doorway With an Unprecedented (and patented!) Level of Safety

The categorized list of uses is the primary guide map to the HoloBarre's vast abilities.

Philosophical issues concerning fitness, health, and nutrition are critical to making

---

biceps curl, what geometric form has the light of the flashlight described? It should describe an *arc*. From your perspective, it would look like a backward "C."

Here's where you get duped. Too many of these machines have pulleys that require every "curling" movement*—biceps curl, triceps

---

*Consult any good book on weight lifting for illustrations of these movements.

HoloBarre can do 99% of the exercises that 99% of the population needs.

It can accomplish this with instant convenience, shifting from exercise to exercise in SECONDS, sometimes SPLIT seconds, with enormous load bearing capacity and safety, with no stress on the doorjamb or hallway, or whereever it is attached.

The HoloBarre claims following:

For the remaining 1% of the exercises for the remaining 1% of the population, attachments exist which allow the HoloBarre System to effectively *DUPLICATE THE FUNCTION OF VIRTUALLY EVERY EXERCISE MACHINE KNOWN TO MAN* (and then some), as well as supporting semi-exotic equipment such as heavy boxing bags, speed bags, and other sport-specific equipment.

The free-standing version accommodates full gymnastic apparatus, as well as extensive applications to physical therapy and rehab.

How and Why these claims can be made

Why hasn't other equipment been made that could make these claims?

The HoloBarre can make the extraordinary claims made on the previous screens because it fully utilizes basic but very powerful principles that have been largely ignored, essentially because "higher-tech" solutions to exercise are more marketable and therefore more profitable. Any undergraduate science or engineering student is quite familiar with these principles, but because these principles are a little subtle and therefore not so easily marketable in the way the products curl, butterfly, pullover, front deltoid raise, side lateral deltoid raise, etc.—*should* describe an arc when performed properly. But they *don't* when you try and do the correct movement on the machine. There is usually a handle, a cable, and a pulley on the machine. When you try to do any movement that should be done with an arc, you wind up doing a movement that is almost a straight line. This dramatically reduces the resistance, ROM, and intensity of the exercise. You are getting cheated. Only free weights allow the correct movement as intended, given the way your body is built. Soloflex® shows a guy trying to do a bicep curl. Where his hands should curl in an arc form, up and out from his thighs and then back toward his upper chest, what he does (to accommodate the limitations of the Soloflex® machine) is bend his upper body, then pull his elbows along his sides until they are behind him, and his hands simply move straight up almost touching the front part of his body. If he had a flashlight in his hand, what you would see that light describe as it moved would be very close to the letter "I," basically a movement that is straight up and down, and not the correct form—the arc. That is *not* the way to do a biceps curl, or any of the many arc-form movements. Have you ever heard any manufacturer tell you that his/her machine actually *constricts* your natural body movements and makes your workout much *less* effective? Not a chance.

My advice to you is not to waste your money on any of those machines for they are not nearly as effective as using free weights—which allow complete ROM and the correct, biomechanical freedom of movement that corresponds exactly to the way your limbs and joints were intended to move.

It appears to me that the inventors of these machines are more interested in profits than results. I think you'd agree with that statement.

I will just warn you again that you do not know who is at the other end of an ad, what the dangers of the product are, and what results (if any) have been scientifically proven. I do believe that at this point, you are probably at least halfway to becoming totally independent in your ability to keep from being duped by any health/fitness huckster. Take a few moments and feel good about that.

VIPS

Any piece of exercise that limits frequency intensity duration, range of motion, and increasing resistance, individually and interdependently, cannot be as effective as free weights, regardless of the hype and expense.

No abdominal machine can do as much for both your abdominal and lumbar-sacral (lower back) muscles than the standard sit-up. You need to work both. If you are unable to do sit-ups, you should be under a physician's care, and not trying to self-cure by using an abdominal machine.

Any ad that touts great benefits, especially weight loss and fitness in a very short period of time, and also touts its product as "easy," "fast," etc., is not telling you the truth. By its nature, the human body must be worked harder and harder for you to increase your strength, fitness, and muscular size.

Hard, vigorous exercise does damage your muscles, but that damage is repaired by the body, usually within forty-eight hours—if you give it sufficient rest and eat a nutritious diet—and the muscles have then become slightly larger and stronger.

Machines that use bands (rubberized, metallic, etc.) start you in the movement where the resistance is very small. It's only when you have nearly completed the movement in one direction that the higher resistances come into play. Essentially, well over half your movement is against such a light resistance as to be wasted.

Don't waste your money on any machine that doesn't allow a full complement of arc-type movements.

The next chapter is not just about shoes, sox, and "sweats." At first blush, you might think what follows to be correctly listed as "equipment," but exercise apparel includes anything you can wear, what is a part of what you wear, or is attached to your body. What you can "wear" includes what can be pulled on, pulled over, strapped, stuck, wrapped, tied, and belted on to your body. Sounds kinky to me. This would be funny if there weren't serious consequences. At least one of the types of the pieces of "apparel" has been known to kill and cause miscarriages.

NOTES

1. Soloflex® ad for Soloflex®. Internet ad printed from address: http://www.soloflex.com/SlflxCalloutPage.html [15 May 1999], p. 1 of 2.

2. Holobarre™ ad for Holobarre System™. Internet ad printed from address: http://holobarre.com [6 May 1999], pp. 3 of 4 and 2 of 8.

9 APPAREL
Is It Just for Show?

What do the following items of apparel have in common: eyeglass frames, head sweatbands, shoes, gloves, earrings, necklaces, as well as wraps for hands, feet, ankles, waist, back, and elbows? Answer: They have all been made with the current, hot health item in them—magnets.

According to Quackwatch.com, the use of magnets in what is called magnet therapy is often touted as a cure for cancer, migraine headaches, sciatica, arthritis, carpal tunnel syndrome, tennis elbow, little league elbow, bunions, and assorted pains and soreness in the head, neck, shoulder, back, waist, leg (knee, ankle, and foot), not to mention allergies, heart disease, ulcers, bursitis, dysentery, diarrhea, urinary infection, gallstones, kidney stones, auto-immune illness, neuro-degenerative diseases, liver disease, and a host of other ailments.

We are now being assaulted by ads that show people walking out of a shoe store (apparently having just purchased some insoles containing magnets) and these smiling, perky people are claiming that the pains in their legs, backs, and necks are *totally gone*. Other ads tout similar "miracle" cures.

Since these ads are so prevalent, there must be something to them, right? *Wrong*. The primary basis for these claims comes from a study conducted at the Baylor College of Medicine, reported in 1997 in the *Annals of Physical and Rehabilitative Medicine*. The study provides no legitimate basis for the claims made by magnet advertisers. In fact, the authors of the study admit it was only a pilot study, which is done to determine if it even makes sense to do larger, more definitive studies. In addition, there were problems with the study itself. Though the subjects were supposed to be randomly selected, women outnumbered the men by a two-to-one margin, which raises a serious question as to whether men or women happened to be more responsive to the placebo treatment, which could skew the results. There was only one brief exposure to the magnet and the placebo, and not systematic follow-up to determine if any relief was more than temporary. The researchers did not measure the actual amount of pressure exerted by the objects at the "trigger point" (the point where pain was perceived) before and after the study. Other studies have shown no significant pain reduction in other areas or for other conditions.

One company by the name of Pain Stops Here! in (I love this name) Baiting Hollow, New York, was even selling "magnetized water." Dear readers, you cannot magnetize water. In 1999 the Federal Trade Commission nailed this company for making those and a host of other unsubstantiated claims. The FTC got a consent agreement barring the company from making these unsubstantiated claims. If anything, water molecules are slightly repelled, not attracted, by magnets. They cannot hold any magnetic charge.

There is a cable TV ad making the rounds for Sobakawa Magnetic Insoles. I viewed it on Times-Warner Cable channel 38, in the Atlanta area, at 8:25 A.M. on 12 July 1999 (shows you what I did for kicks on my birthday). These insoles were claimed to be ". . . clinically proven to relieve pain in your feet, legs, back, and neck." The ad continued with the plea, "You have nothing to lose but your pain!" And, get this, the ad claimed a pair of insoles was ". . . an eighty-dollar value for only twenty-nine ninety-five. Call now and get a second pair free!" The ad was replete with the obligatory testimonials. I guess they couldn't hack it at Lourdes. The entire essence of the ad was unfounded and unproven. Don't waste your money, folks.

What other, legitimate studies have shown is that the magnets being produced by these hucksters are too weak to provide a magnetic field that penetrates the skin far enough to be of any therapeutic value. In some cases, the "magnets" are complete fakes that exert no magnetic force whatsoever.

While there are numerous differences in the magnets made for these phony cures versus those with some therapeutic value, the primary difference is that the hucksters' magnets do not move and the magnetic field they generate does not move (they remain stationary on your body and, therefore, the magnetic field also remains stationary. In legitimate therapy, a technician moves the magnets and thus, the magnetic field). We call this a "permanent magnet with a static field." The hucksters have tried to update the old "magnetic therapy" with a newer phrase, "biomagnetic therapy," which, they claim, is "One of the newest therapies to be introduced to the western world from the field of Oriental Medicine." See the ad for Alternative Healthy Stores at Internet address: http://st4.yahoo.com/racer/noname2.html. These people don't read history. In the United States alone, biomagnetic therapy has been attempted for at least *one hundred years*. The founder of the Christian Science movement, Mary Baker Eddy; the founder of chiropractic, Daniel David Palmer; and others used it—without success.

In proper "clinical application" the magnets move as well as the field (a technician moves the magnets across the patient's body). We call this a "pulsed-field dynamic magnet." These latter magnets have been used successfully in forcing bone growth (postfracture). When the magnet is moved over an area of the body, it causes the bones and tissue underneath to move, which causes them to grow and reattach fibers with the bones and tissues. But these magnets and the equipment used with them are quite expensive—too expensive for mass consumption. The correct terminology utilizing pulsed-field dynamic magnets is "pulsating electromagnetic field therapy," and that application is scientifically legitimate.

I know. I know. The ads for the power of magnets are hard to ignore. They are everywhere. The testimonials are very convincing. But these permanent magnets with static fields have been used for over half a century and only *one* study—with just *one* limited application—has ever found any therapeutic value in magnets.

The hucksters are duping people left and right. The power of your newly acquired knowledge regarding magnets is the main force that will force the hucksters out of business. Let's hope so. It has gotten so bad that I have noticed some ads for sleep pads, pillows, and hair products using magnets. Hair products? I'm not kidding. They claim to clean the hair shaft by vibrating the "dirt particles" off of the hair shafts.

There are some products out there that make me absolutely livid. There is more than one manufacturer but the theory is still the same. These products are designed to give you a shock in your abdominal area. If you think I'm kidding about using the word "shock," look it up in the dictionary and, when you see an ad for one of these products, ask yourself if I'm not using the word "shock" correctly. There were products like this on the market back in 1967. At that time, the product (called the Relax-A-Cizor) looked like a small briefcase. When opened, viewers saw a set of three dials with coated wires coming out of them. The wires led to thin pads (about four inches in diameter) which were set in a webbed wrap that went around the abdominal area and back. When you turned on this "machine" an electrical charge went from the box, down the wires, into the pads, and then into the body. It caused an involuntary contraction of the muscles under and near the pad. You could increase the force of the electrical impulse by turning the dials. This machine was supposed to give you a slimmer waist and stronger stomach without any effort. That machine caused several miscarriages and killed people. It was yanked off the market.

Take a look at the ad for BodyVibes® from Thane Fitness. I snared it off the Internet on 29 September 1999 at Internet address: http://bodyvibe.com/bodyvibesproducts.asp?client+250&confirmation+570963. The first words are incorrect. This product is *not* isometric. Isometric means a force is applied against an immovable object. Bringing an essential element forward from the previous chapter—Range of Motion—the ROM in an isometric exercise is zero. With BodyVibes the abdominal muscles must *move,* since they are shocked with an electrical impulse, which causes the muscles to contract and then relax—this is movement! If the abdominal muscles did not move, they could not cause the impulse to be sent into the body, for it is only when your abdominal muscles "relax" that they move forward and downward, causing the impulse to be sent. The abdominal muscles must be pressed against the pads placed on them, otherwise the electrical impulses cannot "jump" across empty space to cause the muscles to contract. Physical contact between the muscles and the pad is necessary.

Anybody at Thane Fitness want to challenge me on how many calories this thing burns (especially after my proof regarding Christie Brinkley, from the previous chapter)? If you look at the next page of the ad, near the bottom, it states, "Studies show people burning extra calories just by sitting there, wearing BodyVibes, and tightening their tummies." Of course, we never see the studies, we never are told how many calories per time period, and there is one other huge fallacy having to do with spot reducing. Unfortunately, there is *nothing* (save liposuction or amputation) that will reduce the size of only a certain part of the body, and you cannot—repeat, c-a-n-n-o-t—lose size *or* weight in just one area of your body. The ad's claim is absolutely false—there's no truth to it whatsoever. Calling this product "The Easiest, Fastest, Most Effective Way to Help Flatten Your Tummy Like a Pancake!" is patently absurd. Given the history of similar products, it could kill you as well as an unborn child.

Look at the third page of the ad, at the bottom, where this "Lory LaGro" claims, "In only 3 months I lost 7 pounds!" Well, in the previous chapter I proved it would take Christie Brinkley twenty-eight months to lose eight pounds (at the calculated rate of 4.13 calories per minute energy expenditure). That means Lory LaGro would have to expend approximately nine times the number of calories per minute—all else being equal—to lose seven pounds in three months, since she lost approximately the same amount of weight in one-ninth the time. That means an expenditure of 9×4.13, or 37.17 calories per minute. If Lory LaGro didn't do that, then she can't have lost seven pounds in three months. You might say that she might have "worked" more than eight minutes (total) per day, as Brinkley implied. Okay, but where is the proof? There isn't any. Don't waste your money on this product or any other product that electrically stimulates (shocks) your muscles.

There are legitimate uses of electronic stimulators, but these devices are actually considered *medical* devices. The medical uses would be for the relaxation of muscles at the site of a muscle spasm, increasing blood circulation, and poststroke muscle rehabilitation. If you looked closely, you would notice that the devices are used on the body *only* by individuals who have the proper, specific training in their use. And it usually takes a physician's directive to allow their use; i.e., the physician may direct a therapist to use a certain device to help alleviate muscle spasms in a patient. These devices are *not* something you should ever use on yourself. You would be self-diagnosing and self-treating. Please, don't do it.

Some hucksters claim their electrical muscle stimulators can even be used as a diagnostic tool, when they introduce some medications into your body. The *only* legitimate and proven diagnostic use is for the diagnosing of cystic fibrosis. Do you want someone who is not a medical doctor trying to diagnose whether you or a loved one has cystic fibrosis?

I don't—and you shouldn't—care how well-meaning or sincere a manufacturer or seller of "public consumption" electrical stimulation machines is. *It is not the intent that counts for anything; the effect (result) counts for everything.*

Over thirty-five years ago, ankle weights were popular "apparel" for athletes. The theory was based on the "overload" principle, which meant that you should perform a movement, like running with ankle weights attached, and, when you removed the weights, you could run faster and your legs would be stronger. Somebody forgot to tell your legs. What happened was a near epidemic of shin splints, pulled muscles (e.g., thigh, groin, calf), and joint problems (e.g., ankle, knee, and hip). And this was just for ankle weights.

At the same time, all kinds of "wraps" that could be worn like a bracelet, a vest, a jacket, around the waist, etc., and filled with pellets, water, weights, sand—and who knows what else—were being touted as ways to help you run faster, jump higher, swing a bat quicker, have a stronger golf or tennis swing, lose weight around your waist, increase your cardiovascular system, or build up your neck muscles (especially the lovely and talented sternocleidomastoids). There were flaws in the claims. They did not spot-reduce anything. There was no proven result as to speed or strength improvements. It was unfortunate too, because I used the ankle weights and a weight vest to try and get into shape to make the Freshman Football Team at Notre Dame in 1964. I made the team, but those "apparel" items had nothing to do with it. I told you my history of being duped goes back a long way.

The biggest problem with the current-day resurrections of those older items has to do with biomechanics. Consider ankle weights: When you put them on, they go on your ankle, which is near the end of a long "arm" called your leg. (C'mon, don't laugh. In physics, when describing force, torque, and distance, you use terms like "arm," "moment," and "weight." In physics, your leg *is* an arm. So is your arm an arm. Ohhhh, don't get me started. . . .) The hip and knee act as fulcrums that swing this rod backward and forward. When one leg is in the forward stride, the weight is swung forward but, since it is nearly at the end of the "arm" (and not near the fulcrum, say, up near the hip), the weight is propelled forward with a greater force than the same, "lighter" foot would be (if it didn't have a weight attached to its ankle).

This causes your stride to attempt to lengthen, but you can only lengthen it so far, so you tense your leg muscles just before your foot hits the ground, just the *opposite* of what the muscles want to do—namely, extend at the greatest distance in the stride length. When you try to force the muscles in two different directions at the same time, something has to give. It does, and it's usually the muscle fibers that tear. The added weight can also cause the joint—the ankle joint in this case—to impact with more force and with the foot striking with too high an angle between the heel and tip of the foot (the front end of your foot may even be pointing almost straight up in the air when the heel initially strikes the ground). Bingo! You sprain the ankle. (Small tip for the uninformed: You *sprain* joints [knee, ankle, wrist, etc.]; you *strain* muscles [leg, back, neck, etc.].)

This information will add to your armor of truth to keep you from wasting your money on any type of apparel that is "weighted."

If you're into the bizarre, you'll have a feast with cellulite removers. For at least a quarter century, since a book entitled *Cellulite: Those Bumps, Lumps, and Bulges You Couldn't Lose* came out in the early seventies, the hucksters have been going wild, not only with claimed knowledge as to the benefits of their cellulite-removal products, but also with respect to what cellulite really is.

The duping process required two steps: First, that cellulite was some sort of "body fat gone bad" (they claimed it to be "different" than your "regular" or "normal" body fat). Second, that their product would remove the cellulite from your body. If you're dumb enough to buy into the first step, you'll buy the product at the second step.

It may shock you (and I do this all without an electrical muscle stimulator) to learn that the term "cellulite" has absolutely no medical definition. Why not, you ask? Because *there* is *no difference between cellulite and your body's simple, ordinary fatty tissue*. Actual specimens taken by needle biopsy and then examined under a microscope showed absolutely no difference. When ultrasound was used, no difference was found. When fat metabolism was studied, no difference was found.

As I mentioned earlier, genetics determines where the fat cells are located; exercise and diet determine the amount of fat in those cells.

What you see as "cellulite" is this: Fibrous strands of tissue connect from your skin to tissue layers that lie deeper under the skin. These strands also separate the areas (we call them "compartments") where the fat cells reside. When those fat cells increase in size, the compartments also get larger, creating a lot of bulges. It is the separation and the bulges that give your body that dimpled or waffled appearance.

The hucksters don't want you to know this, but even if you did, they'd still try and sell you something that could reduce/remove the fat. The array of products is staggering: wraps, gloves, herbal injections, electrical stimulators, creams, sprays, nutritional supplements, rollers, lotions, inflatable boots that go clear up (and over) your hips, pants, sponges, and much, much more. The only thing they all have in common is that they don't work. If there is any reduction in the size of an area of the body (say, the thigh) it is only because of a temporary water loss or skin compression (it all comes back, folks; you cannot "spot reduce").

Rexall Sundown, Inc. is heavily touting a product called Cellanese® that contains an herbal concoction. It's a supposed cellulite remedy, i.e., it reduces the amount of cellulite in the human body. The CEO of Rexall has even claimed that several studies demonstrated a 90 percent success rate. Two problems: Rexall did not do the first two studies. There have been releases, but these were not properly designed. In fact, the FTC has filed suit against Rexall (my thanks to Dr. Barrett for e-mailing a copy of the formal complaint). Here we have another case of an unproven claim. Remember, to be proven, results of a study have to be submitted to reputable scientific journals and the study should be able to be replicated and the same results obtained.

Another claim that industry hucksters push very hard is an enormous amount of loss of "size" after using their product. Here's how they dupe you. Let's say the product is a wrap (a piece of fabric or substance that is placed so as to encircle part of the body). You are measured at several different locations and the *total* number of inches in the measurement are computed. Then a bunch of body areas are wrapped. When the wraps are (finally) removed, those same areas are quickly measured again and this *new* total is subtracted from the "before" total. If, say, your thighs, stomach, and arms are measured in several places, the "before" total might be something like 200 inches. The "after" total might be 188 inches. Voilà! The huckster claims that person *lost twelve inches after only one treatment*. The viewers of the ad slaver all over the ad and rush to throw money at the manufacturer or seller. The result? The consumer gets duped; the huckster makes money.

If you want to get rid of cellulite—exercise; cut down the fat in your diet; and, if all else fails, there's always liposuction. But liposuction is a surgical procedure, and not one of the "amazing, revolutionary, fantastic (fill in any number of false, descriptive adjectives)" products. There is simply no other proven, *permanent* method to reduce cellulite. Even a procedure called "Endodermologie," while approved by the FDA in 1998, is only advertised as "*temporarily* improving the *appearance* of cellulite." Notice that there is no mention of actual *removal* of cellulite. Endodermologie is a procedure that uses a handheld machine having a suction device located between two rollers.

It is supposed to "smooth out" the pockmark appearance of cellulite at the visible skin level. It apparently does, but the visual benefit is only temporary. It only squeezes and suctions the outer skin layers, causing a temporary repositioning of the skin—but *not* the removal or destruction of the cellulite.

Some claims attempt to dupe you by using extraordinary numbers when stating the benefits. I saw a really funny ad on Times-Warner Cable TV channel 44, in the Atlanta area, on 31 July 1999 about 6:30 P.M. This was for a product called the Fuzuoku 9000. Kinda sounds like some snazzy foreign import auto, doesn't it? All attempts at humor aside, it does qualify as "apparel" because it includes vibrators one person wears at his/her fingertips to massage somebody else. The ad shows a woman massaging a man's upper back (her massage technique—finger placement, force, and direction—were all wrong, but most viewers wouldn't know that). While the woman was doing this, a voice said, "A friend can give you a massage. This is 9,000 times better." Oh, really? How in the world did anybody come up with that figure? Of course it's not true. Don't get suckered by this one.

Because of the attention they have received from being worn by athletes, Breathe Right Nasal Strips® have become quite popular. The claims are essentially that the nasal strips allow the wearer to breathe deeper, take in more oxygen, open up clogged sinus passages, enhance athletic performance, and increase endurance during exercise and/or competitive events. There have been several well-designed scientific studies to evaluate those claims. One study showed that, to a *small* degree, the nasal strips appeared to be able to assist in athletic performance, but only where high body temperatures of the athletes (caused by participation in hot, humid conditions for an extended period of time) resulted because of those conditions (see www.sportsci.org/traintech/breatheright/fch.htm). Body temperature causes dilation of blood vessels to carry heat to the skin surface for evaporation and dissipation. In the nasal cavities, the strips are supposed to increase the inner volume of the nasal passages to allow more oxygen intake.

There have been mixed results in studies that were done to evaluate whether the nasal strips were effective in reducing snoring and dryness of the mouth while sleeping. Some studies showed them to be effective; others did not.

However, when it comes to allowing the wearer to breathe deeper, take in more oxygen, open up clogged sinus passages, enhance athletic performance, and increase endurance during exercise and/or competitive events, the nasal strips were *not* shown to make any significant difference.

So, you jocks will not make the all-star team just by using them, but you night owls might find them useful for yourself (or your partner) if one/both of you snore or have mouth dryness. The results are *not* guaranteed.

Be aware that the big push with these nasal strips is for the athlete. Testimonials are very misleading. Even Jerry Rice, a cinch for the Pro Football Hall of Fame and, in my humble opinion, the greatest receiver in pro-football history, was on television not long ago stating that, in the fourth quarter, when other players were getting tired, he was getting a second wind because he was wearing the nasal strips. I paid close attention to the other players. It appeared that most of them (at least around this time) were also wearing the nasal strips. Why were they getting tired and Mr. Rice was getting his second wind? I don't have an answer. I don't know how anyone could create a controlled study to validate or invalidate his claim. Given his incredible performance throughout his career up to that time, I doubt that the nasal strips had anything to do with the level of his performance. What do you sports fans think?

What I do think is that, unless and until the claim made can be scientifically proven, it is unproven. Given the extraordinary amounts of money, job security, and ego that are at stake in major sports at the college and professional levels, every owner, athletic director, coach, player, trainer, and fan would want to use anything that could give any of the players an edge. Unfortunately, I do not know of a single team that is involved in such a study. So, don't get duped just because Jerry Rice makes an unproven claim.

There is a veritable plethora of garments, braces, and wraps that supposedly act to "increase your (part of body—usually a joint or major muscle area) support." When you think about this, it should really be a no-brainer. But there is a great amount of subtlety at work here.

The word "support" has many different meanings. They are primarily orthopedic, tissue/organ, and thermogenic (heat regulation and retention). Orthopedic supports are hardly ever touted by hucksters with one notable exception; that being the "one size fits all" claim. One size does *not* fit all. You should never wear any brace, especially a knee brace, unless and until it has been approved and fitted by a physician or a certified athletic trainer. To do otherwise is to risk exerting forces on a joint where you don't want them, and not supporting areas that you do.

The tissue/organ is a type of wrap that is wound around a muscle (like the hamstring muscle of the leg) to keep that organ or tissue from flexing. A secondary use is to prevent blood flow into an area where there has been a tear of the tissue or organ. More than anything else, it is the blood flowing into an area and causing pressure on the nerves that carry the pain impulse to the brain cause the pain to be felt. These wraps are also something that you need to have a specialist put on you and, depending on that person's advice, he/she may allow you to wrap yourself. It is not something you ever want to do yourself. Make the wrap too tight and it may cut off your blood circulation entirely; make it too loose and there is little benefit derived. And there is not a whole lot of latitude either way.

Unfortunately, some hucksters have gotten into the act by claiming that a tightly wrapped muscle will contract and relax faster than one that is not wrapped. That's a pile of hogwash. It is simply not true. Other claims state that, if you wrap a certain part of the body, it will prevent injury. Not true. It may *reduce* the incidence of an injury (such as when football players have their ankles taped), but nothing short of staying out of the game is guaranteed to keep a player from suffering an injury in a game.

Then we have the garments and wraps that supposedly keep your muscles warm (which they do) thereby preventing muscle pull. At least that's one of the claims, but they don't. Many of the wraps remind me of old inner tubes. Another one of the claims is that you can lose weight because it will cause the area of the body that is wrapped to sweat and—get this—fat will be dissolved and come out of your body mixed with the sweat. This is a case of something that "sort of sounds logical" but has no basis in fact. It's mostly a lie. A *very small* amount of fat will be converted, eventually, to water and will be lost through sweating. Fat is stored energy. The physiology of the body—all of its chemical actions and reactions—gives off heat, so you are burning calories (fat) every minute of your life. The explanation and illustration of fat intake, storage, metabolism, utilization, excretion, and removal would take—

and I'm *dead serious*—three to four *chapters*. Fat removal from the body *cannot* be explained in a few sentences or a cutesy "sound bite."

Here's why: Your body has over 2.5 million sweat glands (also called sudoriferous [sue-duh-RIH-fer-us] glands). They are of two types—*eccrine* and *apocrine*. Eccrine sweat glands are by far the most numerous. They are coiled tubes that have duct-shaped endings (funnel-shaped pores) where they come out of our skin. This is how the sweat gets out of your body. Eccrine sweat is composed of 99 percent water. No fat. These glands exist primarily to help regulate the body's temperature.

Apocrine glands are largely confined to the axillary (armpit) and anogenital area. These glands open into the hair follicles, rather than directly onto the surface of the skin. Thus, as they exit your skin, their endings are actually hair follicles. There is a very small amount of eccrine sweat that is composed of fatty acids. These sweat glands do not assist in thermoregulation.

The stage has been set. The hucksters claim that sweat contains fat. True, but only in minute amounts and it's really fatty acids, and not fat cells. Second, they connect the idea of fat being in sweat to the conclusion of, "The more you sweat, the more fat you lose through your sweat glands." Baloney. When you exercise and your muscles contract, only about 20 to 25 percent (maximum) of the energy liberated is converted to useful work. The remaining 75 to 80 percent (minimum) is given off as heat. This heat warms up your blood. This results in the heat being released from the body by radiation from the skin surface and sweating. Thus, the wrap does *not* cause sweating and it does *not* create heat inside the body. *What it does do is trap the sweat and heat from escaping the body's surface.*

We sweat all the time. If you were reclining and remained totally still, and you had one of these wraps around your stomach for, say, thirty minutes, you could take the wrap off, and it might feel damp, and it would be. But *not* for any reason other than heat and sweat retention at the outer skin.

There are countless wraps out there for various parts of your body that are being touted to dupe you by trying to get you to believe they can "spot-reduce" the area that is wrapped. The most common are wraps for the waist, hips, and buttocks areas. The hucksters' claims are groundless. I've already shown that spot-reducing, save for liposuction and amputation, is an impossibility. As I also mentioned, the hucksters claim that these wraps warm up your body. No way. *The heat is generated from inside, and only inside, your body.* If you want to make your body warm, work the muscles. Even shivering, when we are very cold, is nothing but the body forcing muscular contractions to generate heat to—guess what?—warm the body. This is one of the places where the phrase "all natural" can be used and it is true.

One of the more fascinating factoids I have ever learned in sports medicine is that the body, if performing vigorous exercise, will reach a core temperature which, if not reduced within thirty minutes, will prove fatal. That should stop and make you think.

Please. Never wear those silly, rubberized, full-length, workout garments that don't "breathe." At best, they will result in dehydration. At worst, they can kill you. Not long ago, these garments were used by wrestlers and boxers who had only a few days to "make weight." That phrase means, "to lose x amount of pounds to get down to a particular weight class." The wrestler or boxer would exercise and sweat a lot, the sweat being a result of the exercising, not the wearing of the garment. Of course, the weight loss was almost all water and, therefore, very temporary. In some cases the weight stayed down. Why? Because the wrestler or boxer died, never having the chance to add the weight back. Crude, but true.

And now we come to one of the biggest rip-offs in the apparel business—cross-trainers. For almost a week I have tried to call manufacturers and retailers to find out what the term "cross-trainer" means. Nobody can tell me, but what I found were a lot of opinions, not facts. Here's what cross-trainer really is: It's a term created over ten years ago by the industry to boost sales of athletic shoes. Even that is a little misleading because it implies that the wearer is doing something athletic. Not necessarily the truth, is it?

Here's what the industry wants you to believe: Cross-trainers are a type of athletic shoe designed for you to wear when training for more than one type of athletic endeavor. Does that imply that if I only want to lift weights I can't wear them? After all, I'm only training for *one* type of athletic endeavor.

Also, if, supposedly, I can only wear them when training, do I have to put another type of shoe on—maybe a "specialty" shoe—made for just that one endeavor? Don't laugh. There are shoes designed only for use while weightlifting. I've been lifting weights for forty years and I have never worn those special shoes. Maybe that's why I'm not in the Olympics or in some bodybuilding contest pumped up on steroids, tan from a tube, and stage sweat, trying to smile and look relaxed while my body is strung tighter than a cheap watch.

Some retailers will try to convince you that the cross-trainer is really cheaper than buying, say, one pair of shoes for jogging and one for tennis. Look, when I was a kid, I had one pair of shoes I wore for running, shooting baskets, playing football in the street or in a pickup game of baseball, to school, and even on dates.

What the hucksters are trying to do is make you believe you can run faster, jump higher, hit a ball farther, get in better aerobic condition, and a host of other improvements in athletic performance if you just wear the correct type of shoes. They further want you to believe these shoes have technology built right in, in the form of computer-design soles. And even further, you are told that some jock who endorses them is doing so because he or she knows what brand and style is best for you.

If the shoes are cross-trainers, what am I cross-training *from* and *to*? Is it just two sports? Three? Seven? And, if any of these questions can be answered, then what in the world are "all-purpose" cross-trainers? Does that mean *all* sports? And how many is "all"? I don't think one shoe is going to work for training for mountain climbing, skiing, deep-sea diving, equestrian events, sport parachuting, karate, and golf.

Any athlete knows (or should know) that you train in the shoe you wear in the event. I don't mean to imply that you wear the same shoes in the game that you practice in, only that if you play, for example, football, you don't wear a jogging shoe with no cleats and then change into a cleated shoe for the games. You practice in cleats and you play in cleats.

In the last ten years we have seen the price of a basic pair of multipurpose "sneakers" skyrocket over 150 percent. There is no reason for it except that the manufacturers have created a myth, and we bought into it. I went into a nearby Foot Locker store last weekend (9

October 1999). I looked at over one hundred pair of "cross-trainers." No two pairs had the same tread design. I tried on two different pairs and they hurt my feet. I could feel the tread through the insole, and I mean every design "tab." I also found out that these two pairs were made in China. The clerk sheepishly admitted that the manufacturers, in a drive to further increase profits, are now having them made in China, and the quality is terrible. The price on each pair—discounted—was $69.95 (from $89.95). It honestly felt as if I had turned the shoes over and was standing on the tread, not the insole.

Don't get suckered into paying any more than $29.95. I purchased two pair (one was a Spaulding® brand; the other Rawlins®) at a Wal-Mart in 1994. I still have them both and wear them all the time except during normal business hours while at work. I estimate I can get another three or four years out of them. That's almost ten years for two pairs of shoes and I'm six feet, two inches tall and weigh 225 pounds, so I do put some pressure on the shoes. And each pair cost $29.95.

If you have a real "connective" mind, you may be wondering if "all-in-one" exercise *equipment* could be called a "cross-trainer"? If you did, you are absolutely brilliant. You just connected this chapter with the previous one. Just this day, 15 October 1999, I saw an ad on the Internet for just such a label for a piece of equipment. Get ready. You will be seeing a lot more weightlifting and exercise equipment manufacturers—not just apparel—who will begin to use "cross-trainer" as a way to differentiate their product from the competition. There will be no difference in the equipment. Only the label will change to make you think you are getting even more for your money.

*   *   *

A final point is worth considering, and will be stated as a question for you to ponder. Consider the manufacturer who puts his logo (and in many cases the logo of a team or other entity on his apparel). When you buy that piece of apparel and wear it, you are giving free advertising to the manufacturer and the team. If *you* want to advertise something, *you* are the one who has to pay for that "privilege." Here's the question: "If *you* are the one advertising *someone else's* product, shouldn't *you* be the one to receive a payment from the manufacturer (and the team)—or at least a break in the price when you buy it?" Think of that the next time you get ready to fork over $29.95 for a simple T-shirt emblazoned with a manufacturer's—and perhaps a team's—logo.

VIPS

Don't waste your money on any piece of apparel that contains magnets.

Don't buy any of the electrical muscle stimulators, especially those that are touted as being able to spot reduce your abdominal area. The claims are totally unfounded and older types—but using the same theory—have caused miscarriages and even killed people.

There has never been any scientific evidence that weights worn on the body can improve your athletic performance, aerobic capacity, make you jump higher, run faster, or any similar claims. There is a long and definite history that they can pull your muscles and sprain your body's joints.

Have a good laugh at all the cellulite removers. Then pass on them. Some companies have been fined and others have been shut down because of the phony claims. Remember, there is *no* difference between "regular" body fat and cellulite. They are one and the same.

Breathe Right Nasal Strips® do show some ability to relieve snoring and mouth dryness in sleepers as well as limited ability to assist athletes who performed in hot, humid conditions for extended periods of time. Unfortunately there is no evidence from any of the many, many scientific studies that these nasal strips can open clogged nasal passages, increase oxygen consumption, or enhance athletic performance (except as noted in the previous sentence).

Wear body supports only if first approved and fitted or applied by a physician or certified athletic trainer. Never, ever use any garment that does not "breathe" (allow adequate air

circulation), especially full-length ones that are falsely touted as able to make you lose weight, particularly by having body fat exit your body in your sweat.

"Cross-trainers" is nothing more than an industry-created slogan to sell more athletic equipment. It is a completely nebulous term that doesn't apply. "All-purpose" cross-trainers are even more of a joke in terminology. Remember now, this applies to more than just shoes.

In the next chapter I'll show you how to access literally hundreds and hundreds of pages that tell you who your best advisors are, as well as who the worst hucksters are. Specific names are given, along with many details.

Turn the page and I'll show you how you can get advice—on a daily basis if you'd like—from some of the top specialists in the country—even the Mayo Clinic and the Johns Hopkins Medical School—at no cost to you.

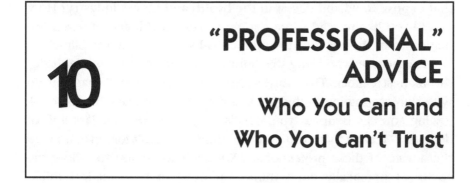

10 "PROFESSIONAL" ADVICE
Who You Can and Who You Can't Trust

When was the last time you looked in a mirror? What did you see? Whatever it was, you probably did not think that the person staring back at you was, ultimately, the very last line of defense for professional advice on the health and fitness industry.

Unless you possess multiple personalities, that can be a lonely feeling. But it doesn't have to be.

There are literally tens of thousands of pages—many of them free—that give you truly outstanding advice on virtually every subject covered in this book. Many of them are in addition to what is in this book. The free pages come to you via the Internet. The hucksters absolutely hate them. They expose the hucksters for who they are—liars, frauds, and people who are more interested in getting your money than in providing the truth.

Let's assume you feel you need more information than what this book provides or, perhaps, you are merely curious about what is "out there" for your benefit. Be happy. What is out there is available—free—and is brought to you by some real professionals.

How would you like to receive—free—a daily e-mail from the outstanding medical staff at the Johns Hopkins University? How would you like to see—free—the very best Web sites (in my opinion) that expose fraud and deceit in the health and fitness industry? How would you like to read—free—some terrific health and fitness information from the best health and medical staff at the Mayo Clinic?

The people who bring this information are truly *professionals* of the highest caliber. These are advisors you can trust. What you do with the information in this book and what you receive from the following sources is up to you. That's why *you* are your last line of defense. We can't force you to do anything. We can't force you to read the advice of these professionals. We can't force you to follow the advice. I personally don't think you need to be forced. I think, because you are reading this book, that you are searching for answers.

If legitimate organizations like the American College of Sports Medicine, the Mayo Clinic, the National Council Against Health Fraud, Quackwatch, the Johns Hopkins Medical School, the Health Care Reality Check, and others, including any advisors you might have at present, can't provide you with the answers you need, then your questions may not have answers.

The recurrent theme throughout this book has been that you get duped because you don't have enough of the correct information to evaluate a claim. And the hucksters want to keep it that way. If you acquire the truth, you have power. I began this book by saying you get duped because you hear what you want to hear and see what you want to see. That may be true, but you may simply not know any better. You don't know that there *is* truth available, if someone would just point the way for you. I don't suspect that there will be many tears shed by the poor, uninformed consumers when they bid a not-so-fond farewell to their ignorance.

While the Internet has provided an expanding arena in which shams and scams can be presented, it is also the same playing field on which the power of truth can be displayed in its full grandeur. That will serve as the starting point for your relationship with your professional advisors, at least the new ones.

As a point of departure, I'll divide these advisors into two groups; those who essentially know and can prove what isn't true, and those who know and can prove what is true. There obviously is a great amount of overlap between the two groups, but it is their emphasis that defines in which group they are placed.

The first group consists of two members: the National Council Against Health Fraud (NCAHF) and Quackwatch. The NCAHF can be found on the Internet at: http://www.ncahf.org/nl/nlindex.html. (There is also an electronic newsletter at http://www.ncahf.org/digest/index.html.) When you get to their home page, you will notice a large number of links. The best of the links is titled "Newsletters." When you click on it, it takes you to a lengthy listing of current and past newsletters. Some of the topics are truly enlightening. Always go to some of the links for related sites. As you go from site to site, you will notice some of the same linked sites appearing again and again. It's no accident. They are just so good.

One of the most valuable—and free—services of the NCAHF is its Task Force on Victim Redress. This task force actually invites people who think they have been injured by some health/fitness product or service to contact them. Why? Because they will tell you if they think you have medical/legal grounds for a lawsuit. I repeat, it's *free of charge*.

The second member is Quackwatch, which can be found at the Internet address: http://www.quackwatch.com. It is run by a physician, Stephen Barrett. I was truly amazed at the depth of research this organization provides. It is far deeper and more extensive than any site I know of currently on the Internet. Some of the information may shock you. For example, if you scroll a fair distance down the home page, you will come to a section entitled "Nonrecommended Sources of Health Advice." Scroll down that section and you'll come to two names that will likely be familiar to you: Gary Null and Deepak Chopra. If those names are not familiar, they've made a ton of money selling books, supplements, appearing on TV, etc., promoting themselves and their wares. I don't know how Dr. Barrett and his associates came up with the information on those two men, but it will surely punch a hole in your smugness if you thought Null and Chopra were at the forefront of legitimate medicine, health, and fitness.

The breadth of coverage of people, products, methods, and organizations at both sites is, I believe, unsurpassed on the Internet. As with all sites I present herein, do go to the other linked sites.

The second group—those who know what is true and can prove it—is composed of four members: the American Council on Science and Health (ACSH), Health Care Reality Check (HCRC), Intelihealth, and the Mayo Clinic.

ACSH is located at the Internet address: http://www.acsh.org. When you get to its home page, look on the left-hand side, under the heading "Issues and Answers." Look below that and you will see a topic heading "Nutrition and Fitness." Click on it. You will be transported to a wealth of information on that topic.

You can pick any topic you want. When I recommend or suggest one or more topics, I do not mean to exclude others. It's simply that there is so much information that if I tried to list every topic, every link, and every topic in those linked sites, the amount of material would literally be as large as a phone book. My recommendations do specifically relate to topics covered in this book. That's the truth. For just the six sites and their recommended links I list in this chapter, I stopped counting at *one thousand pages* of information. I have no idea how close I was to counting the total of all available pages.

HCRC can be found at Internet address: http://www.hcrc.org. I really like this site because it is the most comprehensive site I could find that deals *only* with science-based information on "alternative" and "complementary" medicine. When you get to the HCRC home page, in the center you will notice three blocks of words. The first block says "Encyclopedia." If you click on it, it will take you to a location that lists, in alphabetic order, literally hundreds of topics under the format of Frequently Asked Questions (FAQs).

The second block contains the words "The Scientific Review of Alternative Medicine." By clicking on it, you are transported to the location where you can view the topics and content of the articles in that professional journal. The articles are not overly difficult to read (as is the case in many scientific journals). In fact, some are downright captivating. I let my assistant read some of them and she just forgot about her lunch hour. I almost had to pry her fingers off the keyboard. She used almost a ream of paper printing the text of the articles.

Intelihealth is a subsidiary of Aetna, Inc. The current medical content partner is the Harvard Medical School and the dental content partner is the University of Pennsylvania Medical School. To get to the Intelihealth home page, type in the Internet address: http://www. intelihealth.com. At the home page, I highly recommend that you look at the left side of the page and locate the links for "Healthy Living," "Men's Health," "Women's Health," and "FREE Health E-mail." Pay close attention to this last item. You can get e-mail, either daily *or* weekly (your choice)—*totally free*—by just filling in your name and e-mail address at the prompt (after you've clicked on "FREE Health E-mail"). Below the area where you fill in your name and e-mail address, you'll note many types of health-care information you can choose. You can pick as many as you like. *What a terrific service!*

Additionally, you do *not* have to be a physician to subscribe. At one time not too long ago, that was the case. But studies found that informed patients helped the physicians help their patients, so the requirement to be an M.D. or D.O. to subscribe to this sort of health-information service was dropped. That was a good decision.

Next, if you go back to the main home page, look at the right side of the page under the heading "Visit Our Zones." I highly recommend the sections entitled "Fitness," "Vitamins & Nutrition," and "Weight Management." Be advised that the information you get may be very recent, sometimes just a matter of days. This will help you get better material than the junk that gets the sound bite for the eleven o'clock news: "Plague Hits Ashtabula. Film at Eleven." Then you get a bunch of hot air, but little real information. When you subscribe to the Intelihealth e-mail and/or newsletter, you get no hot air and a lot of information.

I've told several of my friends about this service. I get a kick out of them when they tell other people that, "We get our advice directly from the doctors at Johns Hopkins." It does raise eyebrows.

If getting your advice from the doctors at Johns Hopkins is exciting, why not add the pros from the Mayo Clinic? Yes, THE Mayo Clinic. Get on the Internet and type in the following address: http://www.mayo.edu. When you get to the clinic's home page, look down the left side of the screen until you come to the heading "Mayo Oasis Health Clinic." When you click on that, you'll be taken to a listing of various "Centers," such as "Nutrition," "Men's," "Women's," etc. They're on the right side of that page. Then click on the center you want and you'll go right to it. Take, for example, "Nutrition." If you clicked on it, you'd go to that "Center." Near the bottom is a link for you to click on if you want to get free nutrition e-mail advisories.

If you want a list of excellent *books*, consult the notes from the previous chapter. If you also want to read some excellent *journals*, I recommend those that are located at the sites I have presented above. There are other journals, and I have listed them in the bibliography at the end of this book.

Nearly every medical journal I know costs a lot of money. Anybody can subscribe to them if you have the bucks (subscriptions can run between $100 to $200 per year), but there are a few limited only to members of the organization that publishes them. If you *really* want some journal and it is limited to, say, just physicians who belong to some organization, ask your physician to subscribe. Even if he or she already does subscribe, ask your doctor to order a second subscription. Of course, you better offer to pay the subscription price up front (send the money to your physician) and let her/him send in the subscription request with your home/office address as the location where you want the journal(s) sent.

When you see information on these above-stated Web sites *be careful*. Very often, especially with the Intelihealth site, you will get very current information. A lot of it will be in the form of a report of a recent finding of some particular study. The caution is given because that's exactly what you'll get—the results of a *recent* study. It is usually just one study, not several. Do not make the mistake of thinking that the results of just one study automatically implies an application to the entire population.

For example, if you see a headline: "Recent Study Shows Chocolate Chip Cookies Can Raise Your IQ," first notice that the singular word "Study" is used, not the plural. Second, the word "can" is used, not the word "will." Third, read the summary of the study that will be presented to you. You'll see where the study was done, when it was done, how many subjects were involved, the method of the study, and the conclusions. Most individual studies will state in the conclusion(s) that more studies need to be done. As much as you may want the studies to be applicable to the entire population, they almost never are. They are applicable only to whomever the author(s) of the article(s) say.

Be especially attentive to a study that shoots down a "fact." It may be the first time you'll see the beginning of the disproving of an "accepted fact" that has been used by the industry to dupe you. This happened recently. For a while, most of us were all excited about the potential benefits of antioxidants. But then some legitimate studies found they were not the preventive for cancer as many hucksters in the supplement business were touting. In fact, it was found that smokers who took antioxidants were found to have higher incidence of cancer. The final word isn't in yet, but the question out there really is: "Should smokers *not* take antioxidants if they want to decrease their risk of contracting certain forms of cancer?"

I do not mean to exclude any current, trusted health and fitness advisors you might have, or even infer that you should use the Internet to substitute for their advice. I intend nothing of the sort. Whether it is your personal physician or not, I strongly recommend you write down the specific question(s) you have before you see him/her. And put on that sheet of paper every prescription and non-prescription drug and supplement you are taking, along with the dosage, frequency you take it, and how long you've been taking it, and include any side effects of which you are aware. Some years ago I wrote a little piece for a local newspaper. I present it here to illustrate, in a humorous vein, what may not be a very funny situation as to getting a common understanding of your medical or health condition with your personal health and fitness advisor(s).

"How Long Have You Had This Pain, Sir?" "Ever Since It Started, Doc!" (Solving the Mystery of the Medical History)

"Good morning, Mr. Frisbee. How are you feeling?"
"Not so hot, Doc. I got this pain in my back."
"How long have you had this pain, sir?"
"Ever since it started, Doc!"
"(Grxkqlz). Where do you have the pain?"
"All over."
"All over?"
"Yep. At home. At work. In the car. You name it."
"(Mmmphhh). I see by your medical history, you're a farmer."
"Yep!"
"Do you grow much on your farm?"

"Nope. Ain't grown an inch since I was seventeen!"

"(Ygrglsm). Mr. Frisbee, what part of your back hurts?"

"The inside."

"Uh, huh. . . . Well, is the pain bad?"

"You know a pain that's *good*? Where did you go to school, boy?"

"Sir, I can't help you until you tell me what's wrong with you."

"I already told you that. You sure you're really a doctor?"

"I'm sure. Look, what I mean is, what were you doing when you hurt your back?"

"Throwin' Hey."

"Throwing hay?"

"*No*. Listen up, boy. I was throwin' Hey. H-E-Y."

"What's Hey?"

"Not what. Who."

"Who's what?"

"Not who's WHAT. Who's HEY!"

"Who's Hey???"

"THAT'S WHAT I'M TRYIN' TA TELL YA!"

"TELL ME WHAT?!?!"

"NOT WHAT! WHO!!!"

"WHO'S WHAT?!?!

"IT'S HEY, DOC. I AIN'T GONNA TELL YOU AGAIN!!!"

"WHO THE HELL IS HEY???"

"NOW you got it, Doc. He's my son!"

"Hey's your son?"

"Yep. I know you heard me'n the boy before. I always say, 'Hey! C'mere!' 'Hey! Cut that out!' 'Hey! Where you goin'?'"

"Let me get this straight. You were throwing *your son* when you hurt your back?!?!"

"'ATS WHAT I'VE BEEN TRYIN' TA TELL YA!"

"Mr. Frisbee, exactly *where* were you throwing your son?"

"Out the window!"

"OUT THE WINDOW!?!?"

"Don't shout, Doc. Wasn't so bad. It was only from the second floor."

"HOLY %$#*&%$!!! YOU THREW YOUR SON OUT THE SECOND FLOOR WINDOW?!?!"

"I keep tellin' ya, Doc, DON'T SHOUT! I had to do it!"

"You *had* to do it? My God, man, why?"

"House was on fire."

"Your house was on fire?"

"Yer hearing's bad, Doc. THAT'S WHAT I SAID!"

"*Why* was your house on fire?"

"Didn't have the water to put it out."

(Sobbing hysterically) "Sir, here's the name of one of my worst enemies . . . uh, one of my associates, across town. I suggest you go see him. I don't think there's anything I can do for you."

"Why didn't you tell me that at the beginnin'? Could'a saved us both a lot of time. Uhhh, Doc, you outta see somebody. You don't look too good!"

Please help your physician help you. He/she *needs* your *specific* information to help *you*. A physician is *not* a mind reader. Now you also know why I think that pediatricians and veterinarians have the toughest jobs. Their patients *can't* tell them what's wrong.

****

Fascinating Factoid: Physicians state that from 80 to 85 percent of the information they use to make the diagnosis *comes from information provided by the patient.*

****

I hope you enjoyed that little story and the factoid, and also see the rationale behind the text.

Here's another great tip: If you have the hard copy that relates to the question(s) you are asking your health/fitness advisor, give that person the *whole* hard copy. Why? Because there may be something in the ad/article that will change your advisor's opinion and of which you were not aware or did not think important. The more information you provide your advisor, the more likely you are to get a correct answer or diagnosis.

Here's yet another tip: Take your advisor to lunch. This works if you don't want to wait in someone's waiting room for an hour for a ten-minute consult (and usually it's a lot cheaper). Most everybody wants to eat lunch, especially when someone else is paying for it. This creates an environment that is much less restrictive, and by restrictive I primarily refer to the constraint of time. You'll get a lot more information in an hour than you will get in a ten-minute consult in the advisor's office. Simply tell the advisor or his assistant you just read where people never take their advisors to lunch. You want to do so. I don't know anybody who wouldn't be somewhat honored to be singled out for the kind thought. When you get together, start the conversation out in generalities, but play to the sympathy of the advisor. Get him to start talking about how hard his job must be— the pressure, the demands on his time, the media always reporting the sensational (but isolated) situations of when someone in the advisor's profession makes a mistake. The trick is getting the advisor to shut up once you give him a sympathetic ear to vent his problems. Then you slide the *real* reason for the lunch into the conversation, such as, "Doc, I've been hearing a lot about these shoes and stuff that have magnets built into them. What do you think of them?" You will get an opinion. No advisor worth his/her salt will let an opportunity to expound his/her knowledge pass unaccepted.

I learned a long time ago that, if you want a real quick end to a conversation, ask someone a question that can be answered yes or no. If you want an explanation (something in depth in the answer) ask a person what they *think* about something. Another of my confidential industry sources says that's the key to all the talk shows on radio and TV. He said, "Listen to what is being said. You don't get much fact. You get a ton of opinion. It's always, 'Well, what do you think about (whatever)?' 'What I think is that he meant (whatever).' 'I don't think that's what people want.' 'I think the Packers will win by seven this Sunday.' " It's very easy for people to give their *opinion*, but you'll have a lot of "dead airtime" (no one speaking) if you ask a caller to prove—factually—what he or she is saying. You get a lot of emotion, but damn little evidence. And dead airtime will cost a host or announcer their job in this business.

Doesn't that sound a lot like so many of the misleading ads? You get a lot of words—maybe a lot of emotion—but damn little fact. And the facts are much more difficult—and quite inconvenient—to prove, especially if you don't know *how* to do it and you don't know what the facts *are*. So, how can you disprove something if you don't know the facts? You can't. You get duped yet again.

A favorite trick of the hucksters is to create an official-sounding body whose title seems to imply that the body is really working on your behalf. You might even consider including them among your list of professional advisors. Don't believe that for even one second. For example, there is a group called the Council for Responsible Nutrition. Now, doesn't that sound like some group that really has your best interests at heart? Doesn't that sound like maybe there might be some recognized nutrition experts on it? Doesn't that sound like a source where you can get timely, correct, proven information? Sounds like a harmless, nonadversarial group, doesn't it? It's not.

This group is a "trade group." A trade group is one that represents the industry—not you. In this case, the Council for Responsible Nutrition *"... represents the majority of nutritional supplement sales ... including manufacturers ... suppliers of ingredients, packaging and labeling...."* I just used *their* words, not mine. These people are committed to generating sales—making the industry money. They represent all the key players on the manufacturing and sales side. They do *not* represent you. What they want is your money.

The healthiest foods you can find are in a grocery store. Have you ever thought of seeking nutritional advice from someone who works in a grocery store? If you said no, you are saying so because, I believe, you don't think the person(s) working in a grocery store has any special expertise (as stated previously in this chapter) in nutrition. Why, then, do you get suckered into asking a person who works in a "health-food" store for information? It is because you have made a (faulty) connection between where that person is employed and the person's level of expertise. The hucksters love this and do everything they can to promote and perpetuate it.

In fact, some of the people who are/have been employed in these "health-food" stores may have been guilty of *practicing medicine without a license*. The sites mentioned above, especially Quackwatch, contain links to, and discussions of, studies and surveys of health-food stores. A person would call or enter one of these stores and say that he or she had a particular health condition and could the salesperson recommend something? In many cases recommendations for this or that herb or supplement would be made, and the conditions were obviously serious medical problems. The clerk in the store had no business making a medical diagnosis at all. Second, the "diagnosis" was based entirely on the words of the caller or person who entered the store. Have you ever called your physician and told him or her you had some medical condition and to recommend something? Every single physician I know would ask you to come in for an examination.

TV and radio are notorious for having guests on their programs who tout the latest amazing, incredible, unbelievable, revolutionary fad in health and fitness. And, if you've noticed, it is usually connected to some product that the guest is pushing to make money off the unsuspecting public. Ladies and gentlemen, these media outlets live and die by the ratings. They want people on their show who move the viewer emotionally and the guests want the audience glued to the box to get the latest (false) information. How often have you seen a lead-in having to do with health and fitness, where an announcer tells you the show is going to have just one person on who will give you *only* the truth and the facts—not opinion and unfounded garbage? I have never ever experienced this. I *have* seen and heard people who did tell the truth and did present facts, but they were part of a group of guests who were polarized as to their purpose (never announced as the only guest). Incredibly, the truth tellers have always been put in the position of having to *defend their position*.

The media keeps blabbing about "the people's right to know. . . ." Even if you're not a constitutional law scholar, I defy you to find in any historical government document (the Constitution, the Bill of Rights, the Declaration of Independence, etc.) where there is stated any "people's right to know" *anything*. That may shock you, but it's a fact. Go look for it if you don't believe me. Yet, the media justify their programming on a *nonexistent* claim. It's the people you *don't* see—the producers, editors, and program directors—who decide what you will see and hear—not you. Why? Because their job is not to present fact. *It is to make money for their employer*. And it may take time to find the truth. And that time and energy expended can't compete with the immediacy of screaming headlines. The true bottom line is that media outlets want to increase the size of the readership or their viewing or listening audience to attract ever-larger numbers of advertising dollars and therefore to increase their profits. The price of truth is often reduced audience size, and that's a price most media find very hard to pay.

In addition to media parasites and health-food store employees, I would never trust anyone who is in a health and fitness multilevel marketing (MLM) scheme. Scores of these organizations have been studied. Not surprisingly, the amount of money that could be made in the particular scheme was exaggerated and the products being sold were not only based on self-diagnosis to cure a problem, but also were found to be overpriced, inappropriate, and mostly worthless.

Don't get duped into buying any health or fitness product that comes to you unsolicited in the mail or over the Internet into your e-mail box. I tried to explain in the first chapters that, when you buy something, there's a good chance your name and other personal information (finances, credit card number, home address/phone/e-mail, item[s] purchased, frequency of purchase, etc.) are collected by someone and sold to some third parties. Then, a profile is created of you, and you get on interminable and obnoxious mailing lists that are nearly impossible to stop. So, here come the telemarketers, unsolicited ads, and the like, all designed to separate you from your money. Here's a neat tip: A lawyer friend said that one of the surest ways to stop junk mail is to write: "RETURN TO SENDER: ADDRESSEE DECEASED" on the envelope and send it back. Y'know what? *It works*. And the legal advice I got was *free*. Such a deal.

Never trust any testimonial (whether the ad says it is a paid testimonial or not). You have no way to verify if the testimonial is true or not. You have no way to prove if the *cause and effect* stated by the person giving the testimonial is, in fact, *solely* due to the product being touted or not.

Don't trust anecdotes, the little narratives supposedly describing an event or an occurrence. It may come from the source, e.g., a friend says, "Well, I was listless and I tried (whatever) and I felt better." There is no way to prove cause and effect. An anecdote might also be hearsay—"I *heard* somebody *say* something." A story can get passed on (and, perhaps, on and on and on and on . . .), but it's not evidence for the truth of a product's effectiveness.

I'm sure you have played, or at least heard of, the game in which, let's say, a teacher tells a short story to the kid who sits in the first desk in the first row. That kid turns around and tells the kid in the next seat the story. This goes on until the last kid in the last row is told the story. Then that last kid tells the story that he or she was told. It is amazing how the original story that was told and the last story told are so different. That's a beautiful way to prove why you don't want to believe any anecdote, especially one that is hearsay. You have no idea how many times the information has been altered in its telling from one person to the next.

Take a look at the copy of the letter I received from a classmate of mine at Notre Dame, Mr. Tom Condon (it's not dated, but I received it on 27 September 1999).[1] We graduated together in 1968. "T. J." as he is known, has been a columnist for many years at the oldest continuously published newspaper in America, the *Hartford Courant*. I asked T. J. if he would send me in hard copy the *Hartford Courant*'s policy toward accepting ads for nutrition and medical products. The letter is his reply. I also appreciated his last paragraph. I did not solicit those particular comments. I sent him a copy of this book's formal proposal so he'd know what I was writing.

His reply is very interesting. It also points up a basic fact of life in the media business—advertising is the main source of revenue. As such, you've got to be extremely leery of any media outlet that accepts advertising. Sure, they do it for the money, but what are their standards? I didn't know what a major newspaper's was, so I wrote T. J. and asked. In effect, I verified what I had been led to believe, just as I have tried to teach you how to do. I won't ask you to do anything I wouldn't do myself.

If you get this sort of information, as I did from T. J., you might be able to include a media outlet as one of your professional advisors, but I would do it on a case-by-case basis. For example, I am far more comfortable with ads (at least in the areas mentioned two paragraphs previous) in the *Hartford Courant* than I would be, say, with some of the incredible junk advertised in some weightlifting magazines.

The Hartford Courant

TOM CONDON
COLUMNIST

Larry,

    Here's the deal. We, a fairly responsible newspaper,
subscribe to what are called "standards of acceptance."
With regard to nutrition and medical products, we require
documentation that any claim made in an ad be true. Thus,
if someone tries to place an ad for a tonic that will grow hair on
a cue ball, we ask for a clinical study showing that it
really happens.
    This system is pretty good, but hardly airtight. For example,
we held an ad for a cream that was supposed to take weight off
your thighs. Actually off your chick's thighs. But the
advertiser came in with some kind of study showing it worked,
and we ran the ad. Since the odds that the stuff really worked
were astronomically small, somebody pulled a fast one on us.
Yet, since advertising is the main source of revenue, it's hard
to say no. But we did stop taking cigarette ads!
    Obviously, many media outlets don't adhere to standards of
acceptance, they take whatever comes in the door. So I think its
fair to say this:
    The media is a business, for whom advertising is the main
source of revenue. Responsible outlets, such as mine, try not to
deceive the public, because credibility is the family jewel. But many
outlets have no such scruples. So, as they used to say on Hill
Street Blues, be careful out there.
    Hope this is helpful; the book really has some interesting stuff
in it. I'm sure it will sell.

                                    all the best,
                                        T.J.

ESTABLISHED 1764 THE OLDEST CONTINUOUSLY PUBLISHED NEWSPAPER IN AMERICA
HARTFORD, CONNECTICUT 06115

Just because I like the *Hartford Courant*'s policy, I will not extend
that into a blanket approval of all newspapers.

    Here's a tough question: "How do you know if your advisor is
giving you factual information?" The answer is: "Verify it." And you

verify it by using all the resources I have listed in this chapter. If you can't verify it, don't believe it and don't act on it because you are dealing with an *unproven* statement.

In case you are not aware of it, I purposely selected most of the contents of this book specifically *because* those topics can be proven to be true or false using the scientific method, especially what is contained in chapters 4-9, 12, and 13. The other chapters provide either the foundation or some advanced information to educate you as to how you *can* prove something to be true or not, and this information *can* nonetheless be verified, just not using the scientific method.

VIPS

Be extremely cautious of anyone who is giving you advice who has a financial interest in the result of the advice (such as a lead-in to purchasing a product), especially if that person does not know you, as is the case with all media ads—they are *not* specifically directed to you personally.

You are the last line of defense. You, and only you, ultimately make the decision to purchase the item.

There is a tremendous amount of factual and truthful information available to you via the Internet. And it's all free. Some books and journals will have to be purchased. Use the sources (including your libraries) I present in this chapter.

Take your advisor(s) to lunch. Bring hard copies of the ad/statements on which you want your advisor's counsel. Verify the advice your advisor(s) give(s) you (use the checklist in chapter 14). Then you'll know that the advice is good.

Don't assume that, just because the name of a group appears to be nonoffensive, that the group acts on your behalf. It may be just the opposite.

In the next chapter you'll find out how easy it is for anyone to hold himself or herself out as an expert, represented by a piece of paper and/or letters behind their name. I'll show you what many of these letters mean. I'll also show you which institutions granting these letter designations are legitimate (and which are not).

I'll also explain—with examples—the differences in the meaning of someone who is considered to be *licensed*, *certified*, and/or *registered*.

I'll even illustrate the procedure for verifying whether someone really is who they say they are, as evidenced by real or phony letter credentials after their name.

NOTE

1. Tom Condon, letter to the author, 27 September 1999. Reprinted with permission.

11

LICENSED, REGISTERED, AND CERTIFIED
Politics, Puffery, or Professional?

U nlike the product, service, and person, the title and organization are represented by letters, usually following a person's name. It's extremely easy to dupe the uninformed by simply putting some letters behind your name or claim some "expert status" simply by claiming an affiliation with an organization. If you see "M.D." or "CPA" after a person's name, you most likely will have little trouble in connecting those letters with a level of proficiency and an affiliation with a recognized and respected group. The problem, at least as it relates to the health and fitness industry, is the plethora of letters used by individuals claiming some affiliation and expertise.

Some consumer advisors in the media are totally useless in helping you. You have seen them on TV and heard them on the radio. They're usually put on a program as some sort of consumer advocate and, it seems, they inevitably use the phrase, "Check it out." Well exactly *what* is it I'm supposed to "check out"? Even more important, *how* am I supposed to check out whatever it is I'm supposed to check out? Specifically, what questions am I supposed to ask? When I get the answers to these questions, how do I evaluate them? The so-called consumer advocate almost never gives us this advice.

I'm going to do the job for you that they have failed to do.

Regardless of the letters someone places behind their name, there are three recognized classes of letter designation—*licensed*, *registered*, and *certified*. Don't worry if some of the wording in the descriptions I offer below seem a little nebulous. I'll give a good example to clarify just after the descriptions, and I'll use an example of myself.

When a person is *licensed*, it means he or she has been granted permission to perform certain actions that are *forbidden* by anyone not so licensed. The qualifications for, and the granting of, the license are given by some official body representing the federal or state government. For example, the license to practice medicine is granted by the individual state in which the physician wishes to practice. If a person is not licensed to practice medicine, but does so nonetheless, that person is said to be guilty of either the unauthorized practice of medicine or practicing medicine without a license.

Usually, it takes many years (sometimes of post-baccalaureate education and training) just to be able to apply for a license. And, if legitimate, serious complaints are found to be true against one so licensed in that person's professional practice, it is quite possible that the license will be yanked and the person prohibited from practicing the trade (medicine, law, accounting, etc.) in the state that granted the license.

Further, some health professions and some states require practitioners to complete a minimum number of clock hours of continuing education per year. There are no across-the-board statistics. Most medical requirements are fifty hours, but many professions have much lower requirements.

People who are licensed usually perform some very important function on behalf of their patients/clients and therefore the general public should expect a very high degree of professionalism from one who holds a license.

When a person is *certified*, it means that he or she is a graduate of a specific school that grants a degree designating the graduate as having successfully completed a rather strict curriculum of study, and may well have some clinical requirements in addition to the "book learning."

The certificate itself is the documentation awarded by a legitimate, official body, which indicates a person *or* institution has met certain standards.

The person who is *registered* may also be licensed. One who is registered must also be a graduate of a tough, legitimate curriculum of study. For example, an RPT is a Registered Physical Therapist, while an RD is a Registered Dietician. The "registration" comes from the root word "register," which here is meant to be a formal list of individuals who are members of an organization or association who have completed all the requirements to be registered as a specialist in some area.

Let me give you an example. In my personal situation, I'll pick the most recent (1999) formal designation I possess. I am a Professional Member of the American College of Sports Medicine. I am certified by the American College of Sports Medicine (ACSM) as a Health and Fitness Director (H/FD). It is the highest professional designation awarded by the ACSM in the Health and Fitness Track program. My certification number is 199, which means that (at least as of July 1999) fewer than two hundred individuals worldwide have ever attained that level of certification.

The American College of Sports Medicine is a nonprofit organization and has been in continuous existence for almost fifty years. It is located at 401 W. Michigan Street, Indianapolis, Indiana 46202-3233. Its membership is composed mostly of doctors (M.D.s, D.O.s, and Ph.D.s) whose interest, training, and education is in sports medicine and exercise science. There are over seventeen thousand members worldwide. The ACSM holds an annual convention with thousands of attendees and publishes a refereed professional journal titled *Medicine and Science in Sport and Exercise.*

As for the H/FD, it took me over *ten years* to feel qualified enough even *to make application* to sit for the two-day written and clinical examination. The test is tough, covering all areas of functional anatomy, exercise physiology, human development and aging, pathophysiology and risk factors, health appraisal and fitness testing, nutrition and weight management, emergency procedures and safety, and exercise programming. It's no coincidence that this book contains all of these areas.

In addition to my background, education, and training, I was "strongly advised" to get a number of texts to prepare just for the examination. I either purchased or checked out of the library nineteen titles, all published by Williams and Wilkins, in Baltimore, Maryland:

ACSM: *Guidelines for Exercise Testing and Prescription,* 5th ed.
ACSM: *Health and Fitness Track Certification Study Guide*
ACSM: *Resource Manual for Guidelines for Exercise Testing and Prescription,* 3d ed.
Bloch and Shils: *Nutritional Facts Manual*
Durstine: *ACSM's Exercise Management for Persons with Chronic Diseases and Disabilities*
Franks and Howley: *Fitness Leader's Handbook*
Hamill and Knutzen: *Biomechanics and Anatomy of Human Movement*
Howley and Franks: *Health Fitness Instructor's Handbook,* 3d ed.
Katch and McArdle: *Nutrition, Health and Exercise*
Kendall et al.: *Muscles: Testing and Function,* 4th ed.
Lilly: *Pathophysiology of Heart Disease,* 2d ed.
Marriott: *ECG/PDQ*
McArdle: *Exercise Physiology,* 4th ed.
McArdle et al.: *Essentials of Exercise Physiology*
Moore: *Clinically Oriented Anatomy*
Peterson: *ACSM's Health Fitness Facility Standards and Guidelines,* 2d ed.
Skinner: *Exercise Testing and Exercise Prescription for Special Cases*
West: *Pulmonary Pathophysiology,* 5th ed.
West: *Respiratory Physiology,* 5th ed.

When I asked what should I know in the various texts, the one-word answer was blunt: "Everything." Also know I received no educational credit for learning the content of those nineteen publications; it took six months of intense study to get through them all; and I paid for the texts (over $700), the application ($375), and the travel/lodging/meals (over $300) out of my own pocket. None of it was reimbursed, although it was tax deductible. It was all done on my own time.

And, since I am now officially certified, I get to spend several more thousands of dollars over the next three years attending annual conferences and taking ACSM-approved continuing education courses just to keep the certificate current (the certificate renews on three-year cycles).

Anyone who wants to verify my credentials can call or write the Certification Department at ACSM. You must give them my name. Be advised, you can't just contact the ACSM and ask them for a list of all the H/FDs. You need to give them the name of the person you want to verify. This helps explain why you need to know as much as possible about those who treat you.

* * *

Having said all this I give you specific questions—and tips—to ask if individuals hold themselves out to be licensed, certified, or registered as "experts." This is far more valuable than a simple "Check it out."

1. What do the letters stand for that people are putting after their names? To help you, I have a fairly comprehensive list, below. It's easy to put letters after your name. In some cases, it's extremely difficult to earn and keep them.
2. How long has the group conferring the license, certificate, or registration been in existence? Be very suspicious of any group that's been in existence less than five years.
3. Does the group hold annual conventions and, if so, how many people attended the last one? Most large, prestigious associations will have at least one thousand attendees.
4. Does the organization have any continuing education requirements to keep the designation current? Forty clock hours per year is the industry standard.
5. How strict are the requirements in terms of education and training to even apply for the examination for a particular designation? Most specialist organizations require a *minimum* of a baccalaureate degree and three years legitimate professional experience.
6. Does the designating group have a real address, real buildings, and real people working for it that an inquirer could actually go to see and perhaps get a tour? If it's a P.O. box in Sri Lanka, with no phone/fax/e-mail, forget it.

7. Does the designating organization publish any refereed journals and other publications, such as position papers, bulletins, etc.? The ACSM has its own respected journal (mentioned above), plus it publishes the *Sports Medicine Bulletin* and several position papers that are accepted as "gold standards" in the health and fitness industry, as well as *Exercise and Sport Science Reviews*.

8. Is this group profit or nonprofit? It had better be nonprofit.

9. How difficult is the designation examination? If it's several hours, okay. Mine was spread over two *days*. If it's ten True-False questions, it's a sham.

10. How many members are in the organization? Fewer than one thousand is suspect.

11. What types of memberships are available? In ACSM, you have the Professional Membership, the Professional-in-Training Membership, the Associate Membership, and the Undergraduate and Graduate Students Membership. Plus, ACSM does award the distinction of Fellow to the very top achievers. Most Professional Memberships are limited exclusively to M.D.s, D.O.s, Ph.D.s, and other graduates holding appropriate degrees in a specific or related field to sports medicine and exercise science, such as a Ph.D. in sports medicine, sports science, or exercise physiology.

If someone says he's an LNTGSD (I have no idea what that means—I just made it up), and he's a member of the Society for the Advancement of Mystical, Social, and Snake-Fearing Nutritionists, with a total of four members, founded last year, and operating out of an RV in a shopping mall parking lot, the guy's a phony—and so is the organization.

One caveat: There might be smaller—but totally legitimate—organizations that are just getting started or are highly specialized. This is usually the case when you have a rapidly growing field of science, medicine, or health care. Genetics is a perfect example, though there might *also* be some long-standing organizations in that field (as there are in genetics).

Unfortunately, a person with all the right credentials might still be a huckster. I'm fairly certain most of you have seen or heard of a horror story of some M.D. who bilked his/her patients out of big bucks with some phony weight-loss scam or other phony deal (maybe even killed a few patients) and just sold out for the money. Nonetheless, the harder it is to get a specific professional license, certification, and/or registration, most of those who possess the credential feel that they worked too hard to give it up in the pursuit of money, which is usually what it all comes down to in the end. Thankfully, the near unanimous total of all the professionals I know have principles that are simply not for sale. One of the best ways to spot phonies is to ask for any advice they have given, then compare it to what is in this book, as well as the legitimate groups given in the previous chapter. If it's contrary, you may well have a huckster on your hands.

One good way to spot a huckster is to notice a person who is performing a service to clients/patients and it seems that everyone who goes to that person is directed to buy something that the "expert" is selling. All too often, that "expert" gets a cut of everything sold. Ethically, every legitimate organization allows its members to recommend whatever they feel appropriate—if the need can be proven—but only if they receive no payments or rewards of *any* type (free trips, free samples, etc.) for the product(s) that are recommended. If there is a conflict of interest between our advice and recommending a product, we are told to pick one or the other, but not both.

You might be surprised at some of the letter designations that follow. Be aware that some are for people and some are for organizations. As far as I could learn, all are legitimate, but that does *not* mean the knowledge or expertise the letter designation represents is useful. *Only* scientific studies can prove that. I have purposely left out the most obvious one—M.D. And understand that all the designations in some way relate to the health and fitness professions.

Some organizations may offer a certification such as "Personal Fitness Trainer," but the organization awarding such a designation is not recognized by the industry. Some designations are ridiculously easy to get. For example, you can become a "Certified Hypnotherapist" simply by attending a "crash course" given over a two- or three-day period.

- **ACSM** stands for the American College of Sports Medicine.
- **ATI** is a designation standing for "Alexander Technique Instructor." The Alexander Technique supposedly works by "reeducating" the body's movement patterns to restore good posture and, therefore, relieve pain. The NASTAT is one in this field who has been designated to teach it. NASTAT stands for "North American Society of Teachers of the Alexander Technique."
- **ATC** is "Athletic Trainer, Certified," but the person is usually called a "Certified Athletic Trainer." There is a real "Certified Athletic Trainer" certification and it is noted by the letters "**C.A.T.**"
- **BCIAC** (Biofeedback Certification Institute of America, Certified) is the designation for one who is a certified biofeedback therapist.
- **CDR** (Commission on Dietetic Registration) is the credentialing agency for the American Dietetic Association and offers the **DTR** (Dietetic Technician, Registered), the **RD** (Registered Dietician), the **CSP** (Certified Specialist in Pediatric Nutrition), the **CSR** (board-certified Specialist in Renal Nutrition), and the **FADA** (Fellow of the American Dietetic Association).
- **CPN** is the designation for "Certified Nurse Practitioner." A CPN is one of several types of RNs—registered nurses. It's an advanced designation beyond the RN, and is considered an expert clinician. Many schools, such as George Washington University, have excellent programs.
- **CR** is a "Certified Reflexologist." Reflexology is a pseudoscience based on the notion that each body part is represented on the hands and feet and that pressing on the hands and feet can have therapeutic effects in other parts of the body. Proponents claim that the body is divided into ten zones that begin or end in the hands and feet and that each organ or body is "represented" on the hands or feet. The pathways postulated by reflexologists have not been anatomically demonstrated. There is no scientific support for assertions that reflexology can cleanse the body of toxins, increase circulation, assist in weight loss, improve the health of organs throughout the

body, or that it is effective against a large number of serious diseases.

- **CR** (and **CAR**) may also stand for "Certified Rolfist." Rolfing is a method of connective tissue manipulation, which aims to relieve physical misalignment through a series of ten sessions.
- **CSCS** is a Certified Strength and Conditioning Specialist. Certification is awarded by the National Strength and Conditioning Association (NSCA).
- **CTP** is a Certified Traeger Practitioner. A CTP is a member of the Traeger Institute. Traeger work is based on the premise that accumulated tension from daily stress, emotional blockages, weak posture, and accidents cause discomfort, pain, and reduced functionality and Traeger work can correct the problem(s).
- **D.C.** stands for "Doctor of Chiropractic."
- **D.O.** stands for "Doctor of Osteopathy," or "Doctor of Osteopathic Medicine." A D.O. can do everything an M.D. can do. Consider a D.O. and an M.D. to be peers in the medical profession. D.O.s are *not* chiropractors. They take a regular four-year medical education, and serve a number of years of postgraduate residency, just like M.D.s. The D.O.s do take several hundred hours of OMT—Osteopathic Manipulative Technique—as part of their medical school training. OMT is a series of high-velocity thrusts designed to correct misalignments in the body and is not limited to the spine, as is the case with chiropractors. Dr. Andrew Taylor Still founded osteopathic medicine over one hundred years ago. M.D.s believe more in drugs and surgery (allopathic), while osteopaths believe more in homeostasis— the state of equilibrium of the internal environment of the body. It's more holistic in philosophy than what allopathic is.
- **EL** is the "Exercise Leader," the lowest level of certification awarded by the ACSM* in the Health and Fitness Track program.

---

*Anything that has "ACSM" in it means that the American College of Sports Medicine has two professional tracks. The clinical track is for those who work with mostly unhealthy people in a medical facility. The Health and Fitness track is for those who work mostly with healthy people in nonmedical facilities. Each track has three levels, and each level requires a higher level of education and experience just to qualify for the exams, and each level of certification has a more difficult exam.

- **ES** is the "Exercise Specialist," the second highest of three levels in the Clinical Track program, awarded by the ACSM.
- **ETT** is the "Exercise Test Technologist," the lowest of the three levels of certification awarded by the ACSM in the Clinical Track program.
- **F** is a prefix that means "Fellow." A Fellow is one who has attained the highest ranking in a given specialty. For example, FACSM stands for "Fellow of the American College of Sports Medicine." If your physician has, say, FACS, it stands for "Fellow of the American College of Surgeons." Becoming a Fellow is anything but easy. To attain that designation requires many years of practice in that specialty, attendance at national conventions, authoring books and articles in the field, presenting papers at major conferences, etc. If you see anybody with "F" in front of some other letters (usually limited to the medical and health professions, by the way), you have one who is considered by his or her peers as the "best of the best," assuming that the organization is a legitimate one.
- **Herbalism** is *not* a licensed profession in the United States (HC or CH does not indicate a certified herbalist).
- **H/FD** is the "Health and Fitness Director," the highest-level certification awarded by the ACSM in the Health and Fitness Track program.
- **H/FI** is the "Health and Fitness Instructor," the second-highest level of certification by the ACSM in the Health and Fitness Track program.
- **Homeopathy.** Homeopaths are licensed in three states in the United States. If you see designations such as DHt or DHANP, be aware that these are certifications from homeopathic organizations that are not recognized by the American Board of Medical Specialties.
- **LAc and LicAc** (Licensed Acupuncturist), **CA** (Certified Acupuncturist), **Mac** (Master of Acupuncture), and **DiplAC** (Diplomate Acupuncturist) are all correct designations for acupuncturists and organizations to whom acupuncturists may belong.

- **LPN** stands for "Licensed Practical Nurse." Many legitimate schools with nursing programs offer it. LPNs are called LVNs—Licensed Vocational Nurses—in Texas and California. LPNs and LVNs provide basic bedside care.
- **ND** stands for "Doctor of Naturopathy," sometimes known as an NMD—"Doctor of Naturopathic Medicine" and "Naturopathic Medical Doctor." They are not licensed in most states, but are quite prevalent in the states of Oregon and Washington, where two of their four naturopathic colleges are located.
- **NCCA** (*not* NCAA) is the National Commission of Certifying Agencies.
- **NSCA** is the National Strength and Conditioning Association.
- **NSCA-CPT** is the Certified Personal Trainer (only nationally accredited personal trainer credential). CPTs offer health and fitness advice.
- **OMD** stands for "Doctor of Oriental Medicine." Some Doctors of Chiropractic acquire the OMD.
- **PD** is the "Program Director," the highest level of certification awarded by the ACSM in the clinical track program.
- **RD** stands for "Registered Dietician."
- **RMT** is a "Registered Massage Therapist." An RMT manipulates soft tissue of the body by hand or through electrical or mechanical apparatus for the purpose of therapeutic body massage.
- **RN** is the designation for "Registered Nurse."
- **RPT**, **LPT**, **PTA**, **PT**, and **PTT** (Registered Physical Therapist, Licensed Physical Therapist, Physical Therapy Assistant, Physical Therapist or Physiotherapist, Physical Therapy Technician) all stand for a physical therapist who is licensed and registered to practice physical therapy (or as a physical therapist's assistant) in a particular state.

*　　*　　*

Where the public gets duped is when a manufacturer presents an ad—and there seem to be far more on television than any other media—and an announcer says, "And (John or Mary) is a personal fitness trainer." Closely note that the word "licensed" (or "registered" or "certified") was not used. It almost never is. I did hear an ad once where the announcer said the words "Registered Fitness Trainer." *There is no such legitimate designation*—at least not here in the United States. What these people are trying to do is to get you to buy into their "expertise" and then buy into their product(s).

If I happen to be on television or radio talking about this book, and the host(ess) says, "And Dr. Forness is also a certified Health and Fitness Director by the American College of Sports Medicine," you would have enough to verify my credentials. You can even ask for my certificate number—199. No legitimate "specialist" would push a specific brand name of any product, especially in a paid, commercial advertisement.

The best way to verify credentials is to log onto the Internet and type in the organization—such as American College of Sports Medicine—in one of the search engines. Every single, legitimate organization in the entire health and fitness industry has a home page with several links. They all list their address, phone, fax, and e-mail. They and their members can be verified, especially if you go right down the list of questions I presented above. Any legitimate group would belong to some type of general oversight organization, such as the NCAA.

It is not difficult to forge a certificate and hang it on one's wall. In fact, Ann Partlow, who heads the Certification Department at ACSM, has said that there has been falsification of ACSM certificates by people using a laser printer or scanner. I have heard of one guy who printed out a medical degree from Harvard. Apparently, he got a picture of one in a book, expanded the size on a photocopier, and "whited out" the person's name on it, then used a computer and laser printer to print *his* name on it, ran it back through the printer, and put it in a nice frame and hung it in his office.

You are the one who has to make the value judgment as to whether you wish to verify the credentials of people who claim to have some type and level of expertise, especially when they hold themselves up as experts and use some letters after their names to reinforce the reality—or illusion—that they are qualified to give expert advice in a particular area.

VIPS

If you want to verify someone's credentials, it is best to verify them through the organization that granted the designation— license, certification, and/or registration. If the credentialing group is bogus, this will be found out *very* quickly; legitimate organizations will notify their members and also the general public (via the Internet).

The eleven-question checklist above offers the questions (and tips) you should use when you are contacting an organization to verify someone's credentials.

Note that there is absolutely no accepted title or letters, as to herbs or homeopathic remedies, that is approved by any legitimate entity in the United States to denote any level of expertise (training, education, and experience) in those two areas.

With the help of computer software, printers, and photocopiers, it is easy for almost anyone to create a piece of paper that gives them "instant expert" status that he or she has never legitimately earned.

Stay away from any "expert" who gives professional advice and then leads you immediately right into buying a product that they sell, especially if you determine that that person is getting something of value (commission, override, free trips, free samples, etc.) for selling that product. This is a blatant conflict of interest and reputable organizations do not approve of any of their members doing it.

As you approach—and complete—the last two chapters, you should have the mind-set of someone who is an informed and analytical consumer. Don't be someone who sits around all day waiting to be seduced by all the phony ads. You want to become someone who can approach a purchase and say, "Give me this and only this. I know what I want. I don't need your sales pitch. Just fill my order." Every salesperson loves someone who is waiting to be duped because that person does not know what they want and is, effectively, waiting to be sold whatever the salesperson convinces him or her to buy. The extreme case would be some poor soul who walks into a "health-food store" and says, "Uh, you got anything in here that might make me feel better?" That salesperson's eyes will light up with a big "TILT" sign, especially if he or she is working on commission.

If you can't break the chains of living as a potential sucker, you will forever be susceptible to being duped. With the number of ads increasing at a startling rate, your chances of being duped increase dramatically every year. *And this will likely continue for the rest of your life*. Please, break the chains, get some peace of mind, and save your money.

The next chapter contains information that is both simple and complicated. This is not a contradiction. The question posed is, how can one lose weight permanently? and it has a guaranteed, simple answer. But the methods being touted to arrive at that answer may literally be in the thousands. It is absolutely the most lucrative area in which we are duped. It is also the area where the greatest number of people will suffer disappointment, embarrassment, and loss of their hard-earned money. If you ever wanted to know the simple, unvarnished truth about permanent weight loss, turn the page.

12

WEIGHT LOSS
Can't Anybody Spell
"P-e-r-m-a-n-e-n-t"?

Americans have never been so fat. The *Journal of the American Medical Association* of 28 October 1999 published the results of a shocking study that showed, from the period of 1991 through 1997, that the number of obese Americans has increased from 12.0 percent to 17.9 percent, almost a 50 percent increase. And the study shows that everybody was included, regardless of age, gender, education level, race, smokers, nonsmokers—everybody. Alarmingly, the eighteen-to-twenty-nine-year-old age group saw the largest increase. The U.S. Centers for Disease Control in Atlanta said that the figure into 1999 was even higher—20 percent as opposed to the 1997 figure of 17.9 percent.

I saw on my Intelihealth messages from the Harvard Medical School during October 1999 that the caloric needs of adult American women is 2,000 per day, while it is 2,500 per day for adult American men. Want to know how many calories our economy produces every day? According to the American Dietetic Association, it's *3,800*. No, that is not a typo. We are producing 3,800 calories every day for every adult man and woman in America. Where are all these excess calories going? You know where they're going—into fat deposits in the bodies of our adult population. As a result, Americans have never been so susceptible to being duped on weight-loss schemes.

260 DON'T GET DUPED!

Approximately fifty million Americans go on a diet every year. Ninety-five percent of those who do go on a diet will have gained back any weight loss within a year.

There is one guaranteed, absolutely proven way to lose weight permanently—take in fewer calories than your body expends every day. There are three ways to do this: Reduce your caloric intake in the foods and beverages you consume; expend more energy— through exercise—than you are expending at present, every day; or a combination of the two.

Do not ever, ever, ever consider the word "diet" as something *temporary*. If you say, "I am going to *go on* a diet," you are implying that you are going to *go off* that diet at some time in the future. You want to say, "I am going to *change* my diet—permanently." I think it's also correct to say that when a person says, "I am going to go on a diet," he or she is really saying, "I am going to starve myself for a period of time."

*   *   *

I've told you *what* to do to lose weight. The *how* is something entirely different, and it isn't easy. Oh, but the hucksters love this. They know *what* you want; they claim they have the *how* to do it; and they scream in shrill, greedy ads just how *easy* it is.

In fact, I just received (week of 25 October 1999) an ad from those fun folks at Gero Vita International.[1] Yes, they are the same people who have already won more than one of many awards for questionable claims in ads illustrated earlier in this book.

Take a look at the incredible statement they put right on the front page of their fourteen-page flyer: "200-year-old French discovery makes losing weight *almost too easy!*" Well, if it's *too* easy, it logi- cally means it was simply *easy to begin with*, which, if you've ever tried to lose weight before, you know that is not the case. And this "200-year-old French discovery" is simply playing off on the "secrets of the past" that I alluded to in earlier chapters. It's all phony, folks. Don't fall for their line. Don't be a sucker. In looking at the next page of the ad, it implies that you can eat whatever you want and still lose weight. What a lie. What they are pushing is a product called Chitoplex, which contains the hot new weight-loss ingredient called chitosan (KITE-oh-san). I'll explain later in this chapter what chitosan is, what the claims are, what the side effects are that hucksters never tell you, and why chitosan is potentially dangerous.

I said losing weight isn't easy for a whole host of reasons. There are *social* reasons, such as a specific ethnic group that has traditionally eaten fattening foods. An example would be Italians who consume large amounts of pasta. The act of this eating might have been ingrained in the earliest childhood memories and may be associated with family gatherings, holidays, birthdays, etc. The events that accompanied the consumption of the pasta may evoke a flood of good memories. That connection can be extremely difficult to break. There are the situations of a loving wife fixing her husband birthday cakes, cooking "favorite" meals for him, which may be fattening.

There are *chemical* reasons. Sugar causes a change in brain chemistry. Whatever the sugar is in usually tastes good, not because of the taste per se, but because of the brain's reaction to the sugar. The message it sends out is, "Mmmmm, boy, this candy, this cake, this (whatever) really tastes *good*."The brain chemistry, which controls the urge to eat as well as the desire to stop or not eat at all, is very complex. *There is no "quick fix" from any pill, potion, powder, or program. None.*

The chemical reason can be tied to a *psychological* reason. A person may be overweight and depressed about it, but eating fattening foods makes that person feel better, even though it is part of the vicious cycle of "I feel bad because I'm fat, so I'll eat something fattening to feel good." Then, the person feels bad because he or she gets fatter so the person eats more fattening food to feel better. That cycle is extremely difficult to break.

Many times something sweet is a reward. Boy, is this cycle difficult to break. It usually starts in childhood. The child does something good so the parent rewards the child with something sweet. As we get older and become more "self-sufficient" (we can give ourselves whatever we want to eat), we then have already become conditioned to giving ourselves something sweet as a reward.

You may be familiar with these reasons and could probably state a lot more. What you are usually not familiar with are the *biophysiological* reasons.

NATURAL HEALTH BREAKTHROUGHS

200-year-old French discovery makes losing weight <u>almost</u> too easy!

ALL-NEW WEIGHT-LOSS INFORMATION INSIDE

New research reveals the safest way to lose 20...30...40 pounds or more

● Without deadly drugs!

● Without silly diets!

● Without exercise programs that only make you hungry!

Make Their Discovery Your Own!

If you pay close attention, I'll explain how and why you gain and lose weight and, as an added feature, I'll explain that a pound of weight that you do lose is not composed entirely of a pound of fat. Haven't you ever heard about that; i.e., when you lose "x" number of pounds, are or are not those pounds all fat or something else? If you

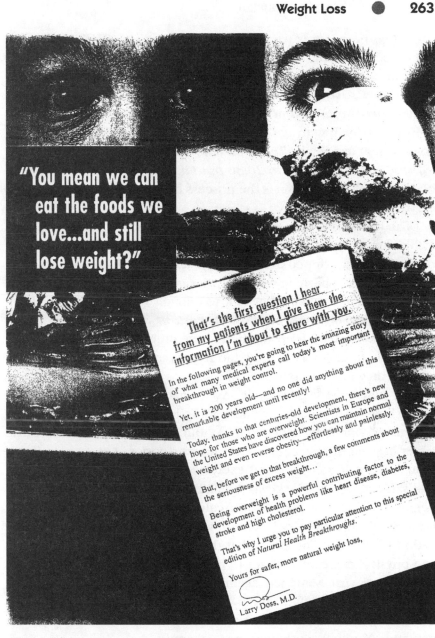

"You mean we can eat the foods we love...and still lose weight?"

That's the first question I hear from my patients when I give them the information I'm about to share with you.

In the following pages, you're going to hear the amazing story of what many medical experts call today's most important breakthrough in weight control.

Yet, it is 200 years old—and no one did anything about this remarkable development until recently!

Today, thanks to that centuries-old development, there's new hope for those who are overweight. Scientists in Europe and the United States have discovered how you can maintain normal weight and even reverse obesity—effortlessly and painlessly.

But, before we get to that breakthrough, a few comments about the seriousness of excess weight...

Being overweight is a powerful contributing factor to the development of health problems like heart disease, diabetes, stroke and high cholesterol.

That's why I urge you to pay particular attention to this special edition of *Natural Health Breakthroughs*.

Yours for safer, more natural weight loss,

Larry Doss, M.D.

follow me, I'll give you the basic truths about weight gain and weight loss. You'll never be duped again about any weight-loss plan, program, or pill if you learn what I am about to tell you.

The most important factor in determining the amount of

weight gain or loss is your basal metabolic rate (BMR). Note it is not called "basic" but "basal." In fact, the definition of basal is, "of primary importance." It's real simple. *BMR is the rate at which you burn calories when your body is at rest*. BMR accounts for approximately *two-thirds* of your total energy expenditure every day. Your BMR slows down with age. It is about 200 calories less per day at age sixty than at age thirty. *That 200 calories a day may not seem significant, but it adds up to 20.86 pounds per year.* (Recall that your body's overall metabolism is the process by which the body converts calories in food to energy.)

The problem is that, as we get older, we also become less physically active, and that is usually a *choice* we make, *not* merely because the calendar has flipped over several years. This reduction in physical activity results in burning fewer calories *and* a loss of lean mass. (Call it "muscle" if you'd like. That's close enough.) *The amount of lean mass in your body is the most important determining factor of your BMR.* You'd better read this and the preceding paragraph again. I want you to understand BMR and how it and lean mass are interrelated as they result to burning calories.

So, here's the vicious cycle. As we age, we become less active. As we become less active, we lose more lean mass. As we lose more lean mass, our BMR is lowered. As our BMR is lowered, we burn fewer calories at rest. As we burn fewer calories at rest, even if we reduce our caloric intake and exercise, we may *gain* weight. Read that sentence again. The key to breaking this cycle is as I stated at the beginning of the chapter—lower caloric intake over present levels; increase physical activity levels above the current level; or a combination of the two. The key is that the *levels* of the caloric reduction and physical exercise have got to be sufficient to *exceed* the drop in BMR. Read that sentence again. There's nothing magical about weight gain or loss. But, unless you know the *how* and *why* behind the theory, you will continue to get duped, waste your money, and get fatter. You will continue to be suckered.

Lean mass metabolizes glucose, the simple sugar that is the body's source of *all* energy. As lean mass *decreases*, the greater is the likelihood of *excess* sugar, which we call (and this is easy) "excess blood sugar." Excess caloric intake leads to nonwelcomed conditions such as diabetes, obesity, greater percent body fat, and a large number of unwanted and unhealthy conditions.

Oddly, your body's fat that is located in the abdominal area is *more* metabolically active than the fat in your arms and legs. Sound good? It may not be. Here's why: This abdominal fat breaks down more readily than other types (areas) of fat, causing *more* fat to get into the bloodstream. Bluntly stated, the more fat you've got in your abdominal area, the fatter your *entire body* is likely to become. Also recall that, in earlier chapters, I said that there is not just one metabolism, there are many different kinds of metabolism. I just supplied more truth to the statement, as given in chapter 3.

Obviously, the hucksters will never, ever explain to you what I just have. As one of my confidential industry sources told me, "The manufacturers and ad makers are not in business to educate you. They are in business to make money." True. But they are so subtle you may *think* they are educating you when they give you a half-truth, which you accept as the *whole* truth, and of course make their job much easier and you become a sucker yet again. Deliberately, they only tell you enough truth to make the sale.

Okay, let's now take a look at what happens when you lose a pound and gain a pound. Due to what we know in the physiology of weight loss and weight gain, what happens to your body's composition in weight *loss* is *not* the same as the change in body composition when you *gain* a pound. That may have gotten your attention. It should.

First of all, a pound equates to 3,500 calories. When you lose weight you are, in effect, depriving your body of some food (either by reducing food intake or using it to convert to energy because of activity—or both). Due to this lack of food, your body *shrinks* because of the bodily components that are oxidized for energy. When you *lose* weight, the caloric value of fat does *not* change when compared with carbohydrate.

Weight loss, therefore, is not merely losing body fat, because weight loss is not composed entirely of fat. In the 3,500 calories, approximately 85 percent—approximately 3,000 calories—is composed of fat. If you ate 3,500 fewer calories in a given week, you would logically think you'd lose one pound of body weight, all other things being equal. In point of fact, you'd lose *twice* the amount of weight—two pounds. Here's why: When you initiate weight loss, protein, water, and carbohydrates are *also* lost, in addition to the fat. Remember when I said you also lose lean mass (and I called it "muscle")? It's also just body tissue. Look back at the beginning of the first chapter when we built a human organism, and see where I show you that organs are composed of tissues. So, muscles/lean mass are composed of tissues. The *caloric value of the tissues* lost in that first week is about 1,750 calories per pound of body tissue lost, instead of the 3,500 calories per pound of tissue that is pure fat. The important point is much of the weight loss is water, not fat. How much fat versus lean tissue is lost depends on both carbohydrate intake and the amount of exercise a person gets.

However, as you continue to lose weight, the composition of the tissues changes, and more and more of it is composed of fat, so that the loss of weight will reflect the caloric value of a pound of fat tissue. Unfortunately, this explains why the first pounds you lose at the beginning of a diet seem to come off quickly, and then weight loss slows down. And that's exactly what happens. Now things get a little whacky. As you continue to try and lose weight (and it *varies* individually, but it *does happen* to everybody), the body goes into a survival mode. The body is not judgmental. It only knows it's being deprived of food, so it tries to conserve its stored energy by reducing its BMR. How much does it get reduced? Approximately 25 percent.

That explains why a "crash diet" may work quickly for a few pounds, but then stop entirely. It also explains why, if you limit your attempted weight loss to between one and two pounds per week, the body will not kick into survival mode and lower its BMR. Please go back and read this short paragraph. If I can get it into your head that rapid weight loss is NOT as simple as some huckster's powder or pill, then I have done my job.

When you *gain* weight, just the opposite of what occurs—physiologically and metabolically—in weight *loss* happens to your body.

There's nothing magical about it. What is great for all of us is that it is so predictable, if it is done without panic. If you just *must* lose or gain a lot of weight in a short period of time, I can think of no better way to fail than to try it that way. And, even if you do succeed, the win is only temporary, and you are fatter than ever, even at the *same* body weight. Huh? What did I just say? I just described what we know in the biz as the "yo-yo" effect. It's the constant up-and-down, up-and-down that people who are continually dieting go through. Look back to where I explained what happens when you gain or lose a pound. Because the *composition* of the pound changes with the speed and direction of the weight (gain or loss), a pound of weight lost will *not* be the same as the pound of weight when it is gained back. This is because the weight loss consists more and more of fat as you lose more and more weight. As soon as you turn it around and start to gain weight back, the greatest composition of the weight gained back, at first, is fat. So, if you weighed 150 pounds and had a percent body fat measured at, say, 20 percent when you *began* to lose weight, you would find your percent body fat would be *greater* than 20 percent when your weight returned to 150. Bluntly, you lost ten pounds, you gained ten pounds, *but you are fatter than when you started*. That's why I don't want you continually on and off diets. You just get fatter even if, ultimately, your body weight hasn't changed.

You may have read something like what I've just presented, and you read phrases like the body's "set point" or "internal thermostat." While technically not correct, the concept is very real and has been proven numerous times in correctly designed, scientifically controlled experiments that have appeared in the legitimate scientific literature, such as ACSM's journal *Medicine and Science in Sports and Exercise*.

Have I just exposed some long-hidden secret of the Orient (or France, or wherever)? Of course not. Any physician, physiologist, dietician, nutritionist, or other legitimate health practitioner knows everything I just said. If you don't know it, why not? The answer is probably because you have been hearing what you want to hear regarding weight-loss schemes. Plus, we legitimate folks are not in business to separate you from your money, but just the opposite. We want you to *keep* your money *and* get the results you want. Sure, we legitimate folks want to get our word out, but we are up against a huge, well-oiled machine where the god is green and anything goes. Our word doesn't carry much weight (pun intended) simply because we don't have the profit motive leading us to the trough of lies.

*   *   *

You may be wondering whether you—and I mean you specifically—
are genetically predisposed to gain weight. I don't know, but your
physician should be able to tell you. You may have a *predisposition*
to be fat, but it's no *guarantee* you will be. In a very small number
of people—I once saw a figure of 0.0002 percent—in a given population, they will gain weight regardless of what they eat. This is definitely a genetic disorder, which leads to obesity. Obesity, by the way,
is clinically defined as being more than 30 percent above your ideal
weight as determined by legitimate height/weight/gender charts. But
even those charts are a little misleading. I've treated bodybuilders,
wrestlers, and football players who were way above 30 percent
above their ideal weight, but their percent body fat was unbelievably
low—less than 5 percent. They were anything but obese (or even
fat). Be aware that muscular individuals may be above "ideal weight"
because they have lots of muscle, which weighs more than fat.

I earlier stated I would explain chitosan. I think it will be around
for awhile before the bloom comes off its rose and something else
replaces it in the hucksters' bag of tricks. Chitosan is made from
chitin, a starchy food found in the skeletons of shellfish like crab and
shrimp. Your body does not digest it, and its chemical composition
is such that it binds with fat. What it does, supposedly, is to attach
itself to dietary fat and pass undigested through your digestive
system, and it almost caused euphoric madness in the health and fitness industry. See the connection? "Hey, here's something that fat
sticks to, goes right through your body, soooo. . . ." So the hucksters
have gone nuts promoting chitosan alone, or with other supplements, as the greatest weight-loss product in the history of the
industry. If it's supposedly so great, isn't there something bad about
it that maybe—just maybe—the hucksters are not telling us? Of
course there is.

Here's the whole truth. In the last quarter century, in studies
using both animals and humans, chitosan has shown some slight—
and I do mean slight—ability to lower cholesterol and body weight.
Of course, the greedy people don't care that the effect is slight, they
just want the proven connection of "Chitosan. Weight loss. Proven.

Yep, that's all we need. Now get outta the way while I make up some words to dupe the public." Trouble is, chitosan binds with more than just fat. It also binds the water-soluble vitamins A, D, E, and K and makes them unavailable to the body. I'll bet that if the hucksters ever learn of this, they'll sell you a vitamin pack of A, D, E, and K along with the chitosan. Also, the absorption of carotenoids (which the body converts into vitamin A) is also impaired when chitosan is present. Not a good situation.[2]

Further, in animal studies, calcium absorption—especially critical to women and older folks—is also impaired, because the lowering of calcium absorption leads to decrease in bone mineral content and, thus, more brittle bones (see Quackwatch.com). Not only vitamin and calcium absorption, but also absorption of certain medications is also affected, because some medications *depend on fat absorption* for their action within the body.

Chitosan also absorbs water and provides bulk. Result? If it absorbs too much water, then you will get constipated, possibly resulting in obstructed bowels. If there is too much bulk, you will feel bloated and distended.

The last point will hopefully drive a dagger in the chitosan frenzy. When you consume foods, you consume not just fat, but carbohydrates, protein, water, alcohol, etc., all of which contribute to your weight, whatever it may be. Chitosan does not bind with nonfat nutrients, so it will upset nature's balance in foods once they get into your body. Nonfat nutrients will be in the body in amounts greater than would normally appear if chitosan were not taken.

Let's have a little fun. I'm going to give you some of the hucksters' most outlandish claims as to weight loss. As you read them, see if you can't quickly figure out why the claims are outrageous. (Clue: You've already been given enough information in this book to figure out what's phony in the claims.) This exercise might serve well as a "proficiency check" (as I learned what that phrase meant when I went through flight training). It's where you are tested, or test yourself, to see if you've learned enough to proceed. No sweat. Only you know if you "pass" this test.

- "Lose weight even while you sleep." I wish I knew who came up with this gem. We *all* lose weight when we sleep, regardless of any worthless junk being sold to the poor, unsuspecting, ignorant public. I just explained BMR, above. The problem can be that we gain more than we lose. That may sound funny, and it's meant to be, but it's also true. Anybody who makes a claim like, "Lose weight even while you sleep" will probably be very successful as a politician.
- "Irving Schmedlap lost 100 pounds in just six weeks." This is a joke. We have no idea who this guy Schmedlap is, or even if he really exists. We do not know if he lost weight solely because of the product. We have no idea when this occurred. We do not know if the weeks ran consecutively. We are not told if Irving has gained any, all, or more of the 100 pounds back. We aren't told anything except what we want to hear.
- "Lose all the weight you want for $19.95." This is a come-on. The cost will never be just $19.95. It's usually an "introduction" price to some plan that may try and snag you for a period of many months, requiring you to buy hundreds of dollars worth of supplements, foods, recipes, etc.
- "Amazing new medical breakthrough. . . ." If it was a medical breakthrough, it would be accepted as such after, and I repeat after, it had been written in a legitimate scientific journal and replicated several times by the scientific community. They give Nobel Prizes for claims like this that are true. How many Nobel Prizes have you seen awarded for some "amazing new medical breakthrough" regarding weight loss, despite the thousands and thousands of claims? You don't need the brains of a Nobel Prize winner to figure out that this claim is a phony.
- "I'm (some famous person's name) and I (some weight-loss claim)." This is a testimonial. The famous person is getting paid to say what he or she says. Some supposedly "famous" people do it for nothing for the free publicity because their "fame" is waning, or to get in front of the public in advance of some new movie or the like. It's called "strategic positioning" in the entertainment biz.
- "This product has been endorsed by (name), M.D." Ah, the

magic letters "M.D." We aren't told if (name), M.D., is getting paid for what he or she is endorsing. We are not told if (name), M.D., has a financial interest in the company that is manufacturing and/or promoting the product. We don't know if (name), M.D., even has an M.D. Bluntly, some people, especially on the Internet, will deliberately set up an operation to deceive the public, make some quick bucks, fold up the tents, and disappear. You better believe this happens, and more often than you would suspect. To be or call someone else an M.D. on an Internet ad or flyer sent through the mail, all you have to do is tap the keyboard a few times. Voilà. Instant credibility.

- "(Name of some food) is 'calorie negative.' " What this means is that some foods have so few calories that you supposedly burn more calories eating the food in question than it contains. You should then continue to lose weight as long as you eat whatever food is being touted. There are a couple of obvious problems here. The first is that there is no food in existence that you can eat that will burn more calories than it contains. Second, if that's all you ate, you'd die in about a month, tops. Your body needs and uses literally hundreds of elements—not just the vitamins and minerals listed in this book. No single food has all of them.

- "This weight-loss product will also flush out impurities and toxins in your body as you lose weight." *Nothing* flushes out your body's toxins and impurities. You always have toxins and impurities in your body. *Always*. Some are absorbed within your body, change composition, and never leave your body. Your body's natural mechanisms keep those toxins and impurities from killing you. Of course, if they are so deadly and disgusting, why haven't they killed you at some point in your prior life? The hucksters want the implication to be that something dreadful will happen to you if you don't immediately buy and consume their product. Baloney.

Incidentally, I wish everybody would have to take a course in anatomy and physiology. Here's why: As it relates to the last little gem of deceit, above, it may surprise you to learn how your body works.

For example, didn't you ever wonder why, if the acid secreted in your stomach can break down and dissolve things in your stomach, that it doesn't break down and dissolve your stomach itself, hmmmm? Well, it actually does, up to a point. Believe it or not, the lining of your stomach is "destroyed" with every meal you eat. In fact, the lining of your stomach is in a continuous process of being destroyed and remade. The cells in your body's tissues continually manufacture new tissue at whatever location they are located.

You may also be surprised to know that red blood cells live an average of 120 days in adult males; 110 days in adult females. They die at a rate of 2 million *per second*, which means that, to maintain homeostasis (dynamic balance) in the body, 2 million new red blood cells *per second* are created. That's 173 billion new red blood cells every day (twenty-four-hour period). The amniotic fluid that surrounds and protects the embryo and fetus is constantly and completely replaced every three hours. The inner lining of large blood vessels renews itself every six months. Both the cells of the stomach *and the entire intestinal lining* are replaced every three days. The outer layer of your skin renews itself every three to four weeks. Most nerves are completely regenerated every four to six weeks. Gums are renewed every one to two weeks. Taste bud cells have a life span of about ten and a half days. The cells in the liver live for an average of five months. Eyelashes, which are more plentiful on the upper eyelid, are shed continuously, with each of the more than 200 hairs per eye lasting from three to five months. The severed finger tips and nails (above the first crease of the first joint) of children below the age of twelve can, and do, regenerate in about eleven weeks. Adults do not have this ability.[3]

In the fetal brain, nerve cells develop at an average rate of more than 250,000 per minute. At birth, a child's brain has close to 1 trillion brain cells. After that, few new cells are added. After the age of forty, one loses about 1,000 nerve cells per day. With a trillion to start with, this loss has little effect on mental capacity.

It is precisely the information of the type I have just presented to you that the hucksters either don't know themselves or hope that you don't learn. It's the overall understanding of the body and its functions—whatever they are and for whatever purpose you wish to apply the knowledge—that makes you dangerous, a person not to be trifled with. When you learn how the body is constructed (anatomy) and how it works (physiology) you acquire knowledge—the truth. That makes you dangerous to those who would try and take your money with phony claims. Realistically, I don't think they worry too much about it because there are so many suckers walking around just waiting to be duped, so they don't lose sleep over the (too) small number of people who choose to educate themselves.

If you want the best book on anatomy and physiology I have ever seen, get a copy of the book *Human Anatomy and Physiology*, by Elaine Marieb.[4]

It seems that every couple of years some proponent comes out with some new diet that the proponent advocates altering the balance of the three basic nutrients—fat, protein, and carbohydrates. What the proponent does, for example, is tell you that you should be on a high-protein, low-fat diet. Maybe it's a high-carbohydrate, low-protein diet. There are only so many combinations of changes you can make. In fact, the number is nine. But the hucksters will try and confuse the matter by bringing in something that is of less importance at the expense of one of "the basic three." An example was the high-protein, low-carbohydrate diet. The theory was that carbohydrates were fattening and so should be reduced. This illustrated an incredible lack of understanding between simple and complex carbohydrates.

Simple carbohydrates are far more fattening than complex carbohydrates. The "creator" of this particular diet had it absolutely backward, but blundered even further when he made his incredible pitch that "these carbohydrates would energize you" so you wouldn't have to exercise to lose weight. This particular diet suffered an early demise, but the fact that it even made it to the "mainstream media" almost defies belief.

*　　*　　*

You read the information from the Johns Hopkins Medical School at the beginning of this chapter, specifically the point that 95 percent of all individuals who try to lose weight are not successful. If you know anything about gambling odds, you would say that the percent of people who will be successful would be just 5 percent, which is— the last time I counted—just one chance in twenty. Let me pose a question to you: If you went to Las Vegas and the odds of you winning at any game were only one in twenty, would you play that game? You might say that it depended on how much you might win, for the odds of winning a lottery are literally in the millions-to-one, but people play it because the payoff is huge. What is the payoff in permanently losing weight? The answer is that there is no one *single* payoff associated with permanent weight loss.

The next question is: "Has anybody computed what are the total number of payoffs from permanent weight loss?" My answer is: "I don't think so." I spent several days trying to find such a list. Everybody seemed to think there was one, but no one could quote me the source. I decided to make my own list. I knew that each payoff had to be something that was both quantifiable *and* beneficial to the body. I quickly composed more than 100 payoffs. The problem with presenting the list is that it doesn't apply to everybody. As just one example, there are some items that apply to men but not to women. Thus, I choose not to itemize the list for the very reason that it is not universal; i.e., it does *not* apply to everyone, regardless of gender, age, current health status, etc. I'm not trying to play down the role of permanent weight loss. In fact, it's just the opposite, for it is the focus of this chapter.

The focus is, and should be, on how you're being duped and how to avoid it. It should also be on educating you about the truth of the phony ads and the essence of what works and what doesn't. But do take the fact that there are literally scores of beneficial payoffs from permanent weight loss and they all belong to you, if you want them.

If I were to write a sequel to this book, it would be on specific diets, exercise programs, apparel—the essence of most of the chapters in this book—that do work and how to do them and/or what I recommend you do buy. The slant of this book has been mainly what *doesn't* work—as viewed by one expert fighting a sordid industry. It's not meant to be negative, but positive, because I show you hundreds of ways you are being duped, how you can avoid them (and why), and how you can save your money.

Now I'm going to show you how you get duped into impulse buying. This usually occurs when you are in a grocery store picking out the items you wish to purchase. You may have gone so far as to prepare a list of specific items. Unfortunately, even people who prepare such lists do not also list the manufacturer (if there is one). For example, most lists will have something like:

1/2 gallon nonfat milk
bananas
cereal
veggies
bread
orange juice
margarine
pork chops
dog food

The point is that you do not put on your list what the label (if any) states as to nutritional values. Here is where the manufacturers get you to buy their product because of what the label says. There are really two parts to the label. The part that most of us think about when we hear the term "label" is the one which lists the number of servings, the amount of calories, the amount of calories from fat, the Daily Values for Total Fat, saturated fat, cholesterol, sodium, etc. This part of the label is usually on the back or sides of the container. This is *not* where you get duped.

Where you get duped is usually on the *front* of the container. You will see big words such as "ALL NEW," "LOW FAT," "FAT FREE," "LIGHT, "LOW SODIUM," "LOW CALORIE," and like words or phrases. It would seem reasonable and logical that if you selected foods with such words or phrases on their labels, you would have no problems losing the weight you want to lose and keeping it off permanently.

Sorry folks, but that is not the situation. The manufacturers have made a lot of noise about how their labeling has made their product(s) much more "informative." They say that the nutritional content of their food had never been "more healthy." They say that their food is "better for you than the competition's" (whatever that means).

What is the truth? The truth is that most of us have no idea what the claims on the front of the label mean. Therefore, they do not inform us of anything. What they do is make us impulse buy—see the box, see the words, react (oooh, this must be good for me), grab it, stick it in your shopping cart. The manufacturers don't care if you know what the labels means. They only care if the wording makes you buy.

Let me give you the inside information and the whole truth. The inside information is that these food labels and the words/phrases used are not something the manufacturers created. They are not something the manufacturers wanted. The Food and Drug Administration (FDA) and the Food Safety and Inspection Service of the U.S. Department of Agriculture created regulations that spelled out for the food industry what terms it could use and the meanings. There was an enormous amount of lobbying to get these regulations worded to the best advantage (read: least detriment and most flexible) of the food manufacturers. I will give you the most common terms and their meanings. Please, as you read them, think back and recall if you can remember whether you have ever purchased something because of a claim on the label—the *front* of the label. I also want you, after you have read a word's or phrase's meaning, to ask yourself whether or not you would still buy that item, knowing what you have just learned. The most important thing to remember is that the food manufacturers *are* part of the health and fitness industry, and your local friendly grocery store may be a lot more sinister than it appears. Read the claims, then I'll explain how the grocery stores help the manufacturers dupe you.

- "Free." This doesn't refer to the price. It may be used in combination with other words, such as "fat free," "sugar-free," and "calorie free." What "free" means is that the product contains no or only some "inconsequential amount" of whatever it is supposed to be free of. For example, if a label states something is "fat free," is it really free of fat? Of course not. It means that it contains less than 0.5 grams per *serving* (not container). The phrase "inconsequential amount" as given in the regulations does have *several* meanings. Confused? In fact, the word "free" may be used with the words "cholesterol," "fat," "saturated fat," "sugar," "sodium," and "calories." If you see the words "calorie free," it means that there may be up to five calories per serving in the container. It does not mean "zero" or "none." Surprised? To further confuse the matter, the words "without," "zero," and "no" can be used in place of the word "free." And you can use the words "skim" milk instead of "fat-free" milk.

So, "free" allows something to *not* be free of something. Baffled? If you are, the food manufacturers are happy.

- "Low." This word, like "free," is used in combination with other words and, of course, there are substitutes. "Low" means that something can be eaten "frequently" without exceeding dietary guidelines for calories, fat, saturated fat, sodium, and cholesterol. Don't ask me what "frequently" really means. It was defined by lawyers.

 If you see "low fat," it means there are less than three grams per serving. "Low sodium" means less than 140 mg per serving. "Low saturated fat" refers to less than 1 g per serving. "Low calorie" is less than 40 calories per serving. "Low cholesterol" gives you two meanings: 20 mg or less of cholesterol or 2 g or less of saturated fat, per serving, in each case. For "low," the manufacturers are allowed to substitute the words "few," "contains a small amount of," "little," and "low source of." Now, doesn't that just make your life a whole lot simpler?

- "Light." This word has two meanings. One meaning is that the sodium content of a low-calorie, low-fat food has been reduced by 50 percent. (Of course, it doesn't say what the base value was, so you can't tell *how much of what* was reduced 50 percent.) In addition, if you see "light in sodium" on a label, it is because that food has been reduced in sodium content by 50 percent. Again, we have no idea what the *original* value was, so we don't have a clue as to what the amount of 50 percent is.

 Another meaning revolves around calories and fat. The food that is labeled "light" must contain one-third fewer calories or half the fat of what is called the "reference food." The reference food is the food that has the more fat or calories and has then been "nutritionally altered" to have less fat or calories. Again, we never know how much fat or calories are in the reference food. Literally, you could have a can of pure fat that contains 10,000 calories per serving (this would be the reference food), and another can (the nutritionally altered food) could have 6,667 calories in that slop, and the can label could still put the big word "LIGHT" on it. What a joke—a real tragic joke that is hoisted onto the unsuspecting consumer.

- What if a product has a label that it is "(number) percent fat free"? Well, that product must be fat free *or* low fat. Doesn't that just put everything in a clear light? No, you have to read, above, what those terms mean to understand what this term means. In reality, the reference value is some percent of fat in 100 g of the food to which the claim refers. An example would be a label that stated, "95 percent fat free." That would mean 95 percent fat free per 100 g of the food contained in the container.

- We've all seen the word "Fresh." When used, it is in the context that a food is raw or unprocessed. What that seemingly innocuous phraseology means is that the food contains no preservatives, has never been frozen, and has never been heated. (Will somebody tell me what "heated" means?) If you think I'm kidding, irradiation is allowed, if kept to "low levels," but heating (without stating what temperature and for what time period) is not stated. To really make this simple, when you see the words "fresh frozen," that means something "is frozen while still fresh."

- How about "A good source of (something)"? Maybe you have seen a cereal box that had "A good source of fiber" on the label. Do you have any clue as to what that particular label means? What it means is that one serving of the food contained therein must contain from 10 to 19 percent of the Daily Value for that particular nutrient stated. Do you have any idea what your Daily Value is for fiber? If you don't, then how can you compute what 10 to 19 percent of something is? You can't and the manufacturers don't expect you to. They just want you to get the implication that their food is oh-so-healthy and you just better buy it right now or you'll die from poor nutrition in the next week.

Seriously, I could continue for at least ten more pages to give you the "official U.S. government" words, phrases, and meanings. All it would do would be to confuse you and make you angry, and maybe not a little frustrated.

The points I want to get across to you are that anything on a label—as to nutritional value—is going to be more of a marketing tool than an informational tool. Further, because of intense lobbying, the references to which values are derived may never be known, so the derived value is a totally useless figure. I also wanted you to see that a word can have several synonyms, so as to further confuse you. And, of course, the metric system is used, which makes the whole exercise one of near, utter futility. It is very important to distinguish between what is on the package (or in an ad) and what is in the nutrition facts panel, which is closely regulated and is valuable. Everything else on the package (or in an ad) may be misleading.

If you want a complete list of all possible words (and their meanings, for whatever good that truly does) that can be used on food labels, according to regulations by the FDA and the USDA, you can log onto a Web site at http://vm.cfsan.fda.gov/~dms/fdnewlab.html.

Don't assume your friendly grocery store is really concerned about your nutritional education. They are in business to make money. In recent years, several disturbing trends have been noticed, all designed to separate you from your money. I know, I know. I stated earlier in the book that the best "health-food" store was your local grocery store. I stand by that. The foods contained there are cheaper and come in far greater variety than almost any store that calls itself a "health-food" store.

My complaint is with the store management, whether located on premises or not. Most larger chain stores with which I am familiar, like Delchamps in Alabama and Publix in Georgia, have local managers on-site, but corporate headquarters are located in a centralized nonstore location.

According to my confidential industry "insider," the first trend has been with the type and volume of music coming from the loudspeakers in the stores. This is very subtle. It is meant to be. The songs played are not soft melodies. They have become raucous, loud rock music. The intent is to get you to concentrate on the music at the extent of any serious reading of labels. The end result that is hoped for is that you will "bee-bop around and snatch stuff off the shelf because one or two words on a label kicks your 'BUY' switch on." The volume and type of music is selected *deliberately*.

Management likes to bring in sweet little old ladies to cook something. It seems like every aisle you turn down, there's another sweet little old lady cooking something. The impression store management wants you to get is that they are doing some great community service by employing these ladies for a few hours a day. Guess again. Store management wants to create scents to go along with the sights and sounds generated inside the store. The scents are usually something that connect with our saliva glands. I'm not kidding. Next time you see "what's cookin'," see if it isn't something like bacon or sausage or the like. It's usually something with a very strong distinctive smell— just like their tactics.

See how subtle all of this is? Most of us would not suspect our "local friendly grocery store" of being a willing accomplice with food manufacturers in bilking the public out of billions of dollars. If you think that is a misprint, next time you go to your "local friendly grocery store," notice several things. Notice in the supplements section how many products have ridiculous claims of the types I have exposed earlier in this book on the packaging. Notice in the cereals and dairy sections all the words and phrases such as "High Fiber," "Low Fat," "1/3 Less Cholesterol," and the like. If the store has one, notice at and near the pharmacy how many "health and fitness products" are displayed, and the misleading claims attached to them. Notice that cigarettes are behind counters but whole aisles of beer and wine are prominently displayed. (That couldn't be a double standard, could it?) If it has one, notice in the "health-foods" section not only the phony claims as to the value of the products, but (if and when you learn) notice also how much sugar, cholesterol, fat, and other "bad" (unhealthy if consumed to excess) things these items contain, and that the prices are truly unbelievable—for example, $3.95 for one 6-ounce "Power" candy bar.

To even further educate you, let me ask you if you think wheat bread has more fiber than white bread. The truth is that is does not. Unless the phrase "Whole Wheat" is on the label, white and wheat bread contain the same amount of fiber. For "wheat" bread, the manufacturers usually just add caramel coloring or molasses to the white bread to darken its color. Cute. Incidentally, if you do see the words "Whole Wheat," the fiber content as determined by the FDA should be at least 1.5 grams per slice (as opposed to one-half gram per slice for wheat and white bread).

The end result is that, while the labeling should be informative, it is confusing. If you take careful note, you'll see that the "healthier" foods are more expensive than the "regular" food(s). Now, that seems odd. If you take something *out*, shouldn't it cost *less*? Sure, unless you're trying to deceive someone.

*   *   *

The number of weight-loss "aids" is limited by only two factors: imagination and greed. If you think chitosan is a new concept, all you need to do is go back to 1981, when the first ads for it began to appear. The concept I am highlighting is that something can block the absorption of something else. In 1983, pills were sold that were classified by the hucksters as "starch blockers." What were they supposed to do? Block starch from being absorbed, of course. And, as lemmings, we all went along with the idea that starch was bad for us. Scientists found out that the manufacturers of these pills had only proven that the starch blockers worked in test tubes. The human body has a different anatomy and physiology than a test tube. As a result, these starch blockers didn't work in the human body because the human body naturally produces a group of enzymes (amylases) that work far more effectively than the pills ever could.

Then the hucksters said, "Well, if we can't get rid of something better than the human body, let's make something that suppresses your appetite by making you 'feel full.' " These products had a variety of different names, but they usually contained the word "bulk" somewhere in the title and were marketed as various types of diet pills. The pills were supposed to contain active ingredients in the form of various fibers. The only problem was that scientific studies showed that the amount of active ingredients was so small as to be totally ineffective at producing any kind of "bulk" necessary to generate the suppression of appetite. What it did produce was gas and bloating.

If fiber, starch, and fat absorbers didn't work, how about something that could absorb sugar? Fortunately for the consumer, the pills that were marketed as sugar absorbers were scientifically studied and found to be ineffective.

The hucksters then as now continue to market teas, herbs, homeopathic products, growth hormone releasers, spot reducers, mental gymnastics, juicers, machines, pads, massagers, and who knows what else as weight-loss schemes.

None of them—and I repeat, *none* of them—has ever been scientifically proven to be effective for permanent weight loss. What you, the potential sucker, have to watch out for are not only "new" ideas, but also old ideas that—by ignorance or design—have been resurrected as "new."

I do not care what it is. I do not care what the claims are. I do not care what the special introductory prices are. I don't care if it has a money-back guarantee. I do not care who offers a testimonial. I do not care who endorses it. If it hasn't been scientifically proven to work—and work across the general population—and the scientific findings have been written and accepted by legitimate scientific journals, and the studies have been replicated, I will not waste my money on it. I have given you at the beginning the three guaranteed ways—the absolute, whole truth—as to how you may accomplish permanent weight loss. Please follow my lead.

Even where somebody offers you a money-back guarantee, would you be surprised if I informed you that a lot of hucksters have *flatly refused* to honor their guarantees? Don't be surprised. It's true.

Last, if you'll note carefully, if you do follow my lead, I will not ever make a single penny from your success. Keep your money and bask in your success. You earned it. I would wish you luck, but luck has nothing to do with it.

VIPS

Americans are fatter than ever before. One in five adults is obese. This means more of us are susceptible to being duped by phony weight-loss claims and products.

There is only one *proven* way to *guarantee* permanent weight loss—take in fewer calories than your body expends every day. You can do this by lowering your caloric intake, increasing your exercise level, or a combination of the two.

Don't ever consider a diet to be temporary. It is a *permanent change*.

Your basal metabolic rate (BMR) is the most important factor in determining the amount of weight loss or gain. As we age, due to the choice we make to reduce physical activity and not age itself, our BMR slows down. Increasing your level of physical activity will increase BMR.

The more fat you have in your abdominal area, the more fat you'll have in the rest of your body, due to the difference in the abdominal fat's metabolic activity.

One pound of fat loss at the beginning of a weight-loss period is less than one pound of the weight lost—water, protein, carbohydrates, and lean muscle mass are also lost.

Beware the "yo-yo" effect. If you keep cycling up and down in weight loss and gain, you *will* wind up with a greater percent of body *fat* at the same body *weight* as when you started. That's why crash diets don't work.

Only you and your personal physician can, and should, develop a specific weight-loss program created specifically for *you*.

Get a good book on anatomy and physiology. Read it. Learn it. Your body is truly amazing. You just don't know how amazing it is.

Beware of grocery stores. Some of the products may be healthy, but management is only concerned about profits, not your health, safety, or education.

Labels on foods are confusing, misleading, and often have

double meanings. It was pressure from lobbyists for food manufacturers on the FDA and USDA to make the regulations as to food labels "flexible and beneficial" to the food industry.

Beware any ad. "New" may simply be an old tactic from the past that has been resurrected to dupe you.

The next chapter will, I predict, quickly rival phony weight-loss schemes as the most lucrative area for the hucksters. It's all about aging. As our society ages, more and more people will consider the effects of the aging process and will be only too happy to hand over their money to anyone who can convince them that they have the answer to aging.

As you turn the page to chapter 13, you'll see that in the title I bluntly tell you that you can slow down the aging process, you can reverse it, and you can measure the change. You can do it clinically, scientifically, medically, and quantitatively. There is no magic to it.

Notes

1. Gero Vita International flyer received by the author during the week of 25 October 1999. Front outside cover, and front inside cover.

2. M. H. Pittler et al., "Randomized, Double-blind Trial of Chitosan for Body Weight Reduction," *European Journal of Clinical Nutrition* 53, no. 5 (May 1999): 379–81. See also Mayo's article "Chitosan for Weight Loss?" at www.mayohealth.org/mayo/askdiet/htm/new/qd990331.htm.

3. Kenneth Jon Rose, *The Body in Time* (New York: John Wiley and Sons, 1987).

4. Elaine Marieb, *Human Anatomy and Physiology* (Redwood City, Calif.: Benjamin/Cummings Publishing, 1989).

13

AGING
What It Is;
How to Slow It Down;
How to Reverse It; and
How to Measure the Change

The claims implied by the title of this chapter are rather bold. I can back them up. Let's get right to the proof.

Aging has many definitions, but I think the one that is most accurate is: "Aging is a progression of changes at the cellular level, caused by internal and external forces, which will eventually result in the death of the organism."

Remember back in the first chapter when we constructed an organism called the human being? In that section I stated that the cells were the basis of life—they are life. Nothing below them is alive, and everything above them is made from a further binding together of cells. Thus, when specific cells fail—even though we may think of the collection of cells as an organ, such as the heart—death will result.

We all age at different rates, and our individual rates of aging are not uniform. That is to say, as a specific individual, you don't have a constant rate of aging of your heart, eyes, lungs, or anything else. They don't change every day, week, month, or year by exactly the same amount as the preceding time period.

Regardless of the rate of change, it must be able to be measured, otherwise no one could make a statement that the rates of aging are different between individuals, and an individual's rate is not constant.

The way we measure this change is by taking measurements of what are called "biomarkers" of aging. A biomarker is actually a clinical test that results in some number being generated that measures a part of the body; substances found within the body; and the level of functioning of body tissues, organs, and systems. What are tested can literally be hundreds of different items.

Forget the calendar. Forget chronological age. The calendar is irrelevant. What is relevant is your biophysiological age—your age of the functions of the cells, tissues, organs, and systems that constitute your body. You may have heard a phrase something like, "Man, he's got the lungs of a guy half his age." You know what? He may well have lungs of a guy half his age. We can prove whether or not that appraisal is true. We can prove it clinically, scientifically, medically, and quantitatively.

You will see in ads and in various literature people referring to the "biological" age. That's not correct, because "bio-" refers to something that is alive. That's all. "Biophysiological" refers to the level of *function* of something that is alive. For example, it does not matter how "old" your lungs are. What *does* matter is the *level* at which they function. Most importantly, you want to know how well they function when compared to the rest of the population. Forty-year-old lungs that function on a level with the lungs of a twenty-two-year-old person is what is critical. In the other direction, forty-year-old lungs that function at the level of a sixty-year-old person are a danger sign. So, the "biomarker" of aging is the function, represented by some number, that tells you how well parts of your body are working as compared to others in the population.

Below is a partial list of the biomarkers of aging you might recognize, at least by name. You may never have thought of them as biomarkers of aging. There are two groups. The first group contains those biomarkers that *decrease* with age. The second group, which immediately follows the first group, contains those biomarkers that *increase* with age. Once you've completed reading the list, I'll show you how to measure any changes in age, regardless of the magnitude and direction of change.

BIOMARKERS OF AGING

Decreases with Age

Aerobic Capacity—ability
Albumin—serum, amount of
Aldosterone (hormone)—level of
Androgens (hormones)—level of
Arm Span—length of
Balance—ability to, continuous
Beta Carotene—level of
Blood—circulating system, density of
Blood Cell Count—red and white, total
Body—BMR (Basal Metabolic Rate)
Body Composition—Percent lean mass and percent body fat
Bone Tissue—begins at age fifty
Brain Cells—not all, but especially cells in frontal cortex—40 percent
Brain (energy metabolism)—rate of
Brain (size)—area
Brain (weight)—seen as shrinking of gyri and widening of sulci (via
    CAT scan and/or MRI)—10 percent less from ages twenty to
    ninety
Breast Glandular Tissue—amount of
Calcitonin—level of
Calcium—level of
Calf—diameter of
Cholesterol—serum, level of
Chromium—level of
Circulating Hormones—in postmenopausal women. Governed by
    hormone secretion of pituitary gland (located at the base of the
    brain), and this is controlled by more basic changes in hormonal
    secretions of the hypothalamus (located in brain cavity between
    the left and right cerebral hemispheres)
Coenzyme Q-10 (aka Ubiquinol-10; "Vitamin Q")—level of
Collagen—level of
Corticosteroids—level of

Dehydroepiandrosterone (DHEA)—level of

Dimethyl Sulfoxide (DMSO)—level of

Dopamine Receptors—brain's, level of

Endurance—amount of

Estradiol (hormone)—rapid, in postmenopausal women

Estrogen (hormone)—level of

Exercise—tolerance and performance of

Eyes—size of the pupil (shrinks 60 percent between ages twenty and sixty [called pupillary miosis])

Eyes—static visual acuity and color vision discrimination ability

Ferritin—serum, level of

FEV1 (Forced Expiratory Volume)—amount of

Fingernail—growth rate of (50 percent between ages thirty and ninety). Toenail rate of growth does not seem to change with age

Flexibility—amount of

Folic Acid—level of

FVC—Forced Vital Capacity—amount of

Garlic—level of

Globulin—serum, amount of

Glucose—levels (fasting and nonfasting), serum

Glutathione—level of

Grip Strength—amount of

Hair—rate of growth on scalp and armpit (axillary)

Hearing—ability to hear loud sounds (tone and voice)

Hearing—especially in higher frequencies (tone and voice)

Heart Rate—maximum (bpm)

Heart Rate—resting (bpm)

Height—from maximum, two inches in men; one and a quarter inches in women (rate of decrease increases with age)

Hematocrit—percent

Hemoglobin—amount of

Hormones (in general)—levels of

Human Growth Hormone (HGH)—level of

Immature Eggs in Female Ovaries—approaches zero at age fifty

Immune System—ability to produce antibodies

Insulin—level of

Iron—level of (especially in women)

Kidneys—size of

Lymphocytes (class of white blood cells)—proportion of subcomponents

Mature Eggs in Female Ovaries—numbers of

Melanin—level of

Memory—short, intermediate, and long-term (visual and auditory)

Muscle Mass—amount of

Neutrophils—efficiency of

Neurotransmitters (e.g., acetylcholine, etc.)—levels of

Noradrenaline—level of

Parathyroid Hormones—levels of

Physical Activity—rate and amounts of

Power Output—amount of

Potassium—level of

Progesterone (hormone)—level of

Reaction Speed—repeated, rate of

Renal Function—ability of kidney to clear nitrogenous wastes from blood

Selenium—level of

Seratonin—level of

Sexual Activity—rate of

Skin—subcutis layer, amount of

Skin—rate of speed of wound repair

Sleep—amount of REM (Rapid Eye Movement)

Smell—ability to detect and differentiate odors

Somatomedin (A & C)—levels of

Somatostatin—level of

Spleen—size of

Strength/Lean Mass—ratio

Stromelysin—level of

Submax Treadmill—heart rate bpm

Superoxide Dismutase (DMSO)—level of

Sweat Glands—disappear/become nonfunctional, especially apocrine sweat glands

Target Cells—receptors that are attached by hormones, numbers of, and ability of hormones to attach to

Temperature—skin, especially facial and extremities

Testosterone (hormone)—level of

Thymus Gland—at age fifty, only 5 to 10 percent of original mass

Thymus Hormones (thymus gland beneath sternum in the chest)—
begin at age twenty-five; zero at age sixty-five

Thyroid—found in the brain

Thyroid Hormones—levels of

Uterus—weight and size, postmenopausal. At age sixty-five, 50 percent of weight at age thirty

Vaginal Wall—length, diameter, and vaginal secretions (in women
not receiving estrogen therapy)

Verbal Learning Task—ability

Vitamins—levels of—especially, A, B_6, B_{12}, C, and E

VO_2 Max—ml/kg/min

Water—amount in body composition

Weight—after middle age; increases until then

Zinc—level of

Increases with Age

Arteries—thickening of

Blood Urea Nitrogen (BUN)—level of

Body—trunk, size of

Body Composition—percent body fat

Body Mass Index (BMI)

Chest—size (diameter, circumference, and depth)

Cholesterol—level of

Creatinine—serum, level of

Ears—elongates

Exercise—recovery time from

Eyes—cataract formation and severity

Eyes—ocular pressure in anterior chamber

Eyes—thickening of and weight of lens

Elastin—level of

Food—intake, amount of

Hair—onset and rate of growth in nose, ears, upper lip (especially in
women, postmenopausal)

Head—circumference, breadth and length (in men and women)

Heart—size of
Lipoproteins—HDLs and LDLs—levels of
Lungs—size of
M-1 and M-2 ("Mortality Genes")—presence and level of
Nose—elongates
Palm Bones—second of the five cylindrical—widens
Prostate Gland—usually after age forty
Prostatic Specific Antigen (PSA)—level of
Reaction Speeds—simple and choice, time of
Rib Bones—until age seventy
Skin—discoloration, elasticity, wrinkling
Skin—dryness and itching, amount of
Skin Folds—amounts of
Skull—bones of
Skull—fusion of (after age seventy)
Sleep—apnea—periods and amounts of
Sleep—NREM (Non-Rapid Eye Movement), amount of
Triglycerides—level of
Uric Acid—level of
Weight—increases until middle age (decreases thereafter)

Let's assume you buy some product that is touted as being able to make you younger. Proving whether or not that statement is true—in your specific case—is what is important. And you *can* prove it.

By having your physician test you, using various biomarkers of aging, you can prove whether or not you have become younger, and the only way that you can do that is by testing your body *functionally*.

Your body is a marvelous organism; its organs and systems are both interrelated and interdependent. This means that, if you decide to do something that is very beneficial (or detrimental) to one part of your body, it will have beneficial (or detrimental) effects on other parts of your body, and these effects can be measured quantitatively. I do guarantee that, if you start smoking, your body will suffer detrimental effects to more than your lungs. Conversely, if you stop smoking, that will cause beneficial effects to more than just your lungs.

What is fascinating is that the beneficial or detrimental effects are the *greatest in the earliest part of any program that changes your body*. From that point on, the increase or decrease occurs at a slower and slower rate. Take weightlifting as an example. You may start out bench-pressing 100 pounds. In the next six months, you might increase the weight by 50 pounds, for a 50 percent increase in six months. To match that 50 percent increase in the next six months you'd have to bench-press 225 pounds—a 75-pound increase (50 percent of 150 is 75, and add the 75 to 150 to get 225). To increase the poundage by yet another 50 percent in the next six months, you'd have to bench-press 337½ pounds. It's easy to see that you simply can't keep the rate of change constant over time.

Here's what I recommend: You and your physician decide what it is you want to do—or stop doing—to your body in the next ninety days. Have a number of your biomarkers tested before you start or stop whatever you want to do (this is called a "pretest"). At the end of ninety days, have the same tests done once more (this is called the "posttest"). Compare the two scores and note the changes. If you look at the list of biomarkers of aging I presented above, you can see which direction the numbers should go (increase or decrease) as you age. If the numbers have gone the opposite way in that ninety-day period, you have just proven that, at least for those areas tested, you have become measurably younger. If you keep repeating the tests at ninety-day intervals, you can also see if the rate of change is speeding up or slowing down. Read this closely: *What you have just proven is whether or not you have slowed down or even reversed the rate of aging*. Unfortunately, you may also learn if you have increased your rate of aging. It all depends on the scores.

An obvious question is: "Which biomarkers of aging should I pick?"

To answer your question, first refer to chapter 2. There I said that for a study to be scientifically valid, we needed an N-size of at least thirty (thirty is the minimum number required by the laws of statistical methodology to attain the highest level of scientific valid). Pick at least thirty biomarkers. Second, it is a good idea to spread them across the spectrum of physiology of your body. You don't want thirty tests all done just on your vision. Let me tell you what I would suggest.

In 1988, when I founded the National Center for Sports Medicine, I created the L.I.F.E. TEST™ ("L.I.F.E." is an acronym for "Longevity Indicator Functional Examination"). It took more than two years to create. What I did was to look at literally hundreds of biomarkers of aging and select a total of forty-five, based on fourteen different parameters (or requirements, if you will). I took the tests and placed them into eleven different groups, according to function. What I came up with was a series of eleven groups of forty-five clinical tests, measurements, and examinations that, when taken collectively, determine a person's biophysiological age—the true age. Here are those groups and tests that compose the L.I.F.E. TEST™. The groups are in bold print; the individual biomarkers are underneath each group title. The units of measure are in parentheses following the individual test.

1. **Body Composition**
   Body Mass Index (BMI) (decimal)
   Percent Body Fat (percent)
   Skin Elasticity (seconds)—how long it takes for skin to resume
      its original shape after being pinched

2. **Cardiovascular**
   Resting Heart Rate (beats per minute)
   Maximum Heart Rate (beats per minute)
   Resting Blood Pressure
      —Systolic (mmHg)—contraction pressure in the heart's
         ventricles
      —Diastolic (mmHg)—pressure of the heart's ventricles
         during relocation between contractions

3. **Pulmonary/Respiratory**
   VO_2 Max (mg/kg/min)—maximum oxygen uptake
   Submax Treadmill (heartbeats per minute)
   Forced Expiratory Volume (FEV_1) (liters of oxygen expelled
      from the lungs in one second)
   Forced Vital Capacity (FVC) (liters)—amount of oxygen
      expelled from lungs for as long as patient is able to exhale
      continuously

4. **Coronary Heart Function**

Serum Total Cholesterol (mg/dl)

High-Density Lipoproteins (HDLs) (mg/dl)—a compound that has the greatest percentage of protein to lipids (fats) and cholesterol. Also called "good cholesterol."

Low-Density Lipoproteins (LDLs) (mg/dl)—a compound that has the lowest percentage of protein to lipids (fats) and cholesterol. Also called "bad cholesterol."

Triglycerides (mg/dl)—the most plentiful of all fats found in the body. These constitute the major storage form of fat in adipose (fat) cells.

5. **Renal Function**

Uric Acid (mg/dl)

Creatinine Clearance (ml/min)—the rate of excretion of the end product of creatinine from the kidneys

Blood Urea Nitrogen (BUN) (mg/dl)—another measure of kidney function, showing the amount of nitrogen in the blood in the form of urea

6. **Blood Chemistry**

Red Blood Cells (RBC) (millions/mcl)

White Blood Cells (WBC) (thousands/mcl)

Serum Ferritin (mg/dl)—amount of iron in blood

Hematocrit (percent)—the percentage of red blood cells to total blood volume

Fasting *or* Nonfasting Glucose (mg/dl)—amount of sugar in the blood

Serum Hemoglobin (mg/dl)—the oxygen-transporting component of red blood cells

Serum Globulin (mg/dl)—the fraction of the blood serum with which antibodies are associated

Serum Albumin (mg/dl)—the most abundant blood protein

Dehydroepiandrosterone (DHEA) (mcg/ml)—an androgenic (causing muscularization) substance. It is a hormone.

7. **Central Nervous System**

Simple Reaction Speed (inches)—using a 36-inch ruler, this tests the ability of the patient to reach out and grab the ruler after it is dropped. The inch scale on the ruler determines the score (the higher up the ruler it is grabbed, the slower is the reaction speed).

Choice Reaction Speed (inches)—using two 36-inch rulers, only one is dropped. Same scoring mechanism as for simple reaction speed.

Repeated Action Speed (number in three seconds)—number of times the patient can tap a pencil or pen point on a paper.

Balance (seconds)—length of time the patient can balance on one leg with eyes closed

Memory Span

—Simple Memory (number correct)—determination of ability to recall correctly a seven-digit number in correct sequence

—Recognition (number correct)—determination of ability to recall correctly seven words embedded in a group of twenty-one words

—Recognition/Recall (number correct)—determination of ability to recall correctly a given number of shapes, whether numbers were within each shape and number of lines connecting each shape

8. **Strength/Flexibility**

Sit and Reach (inches)

Grip Strength (kg)

Strength/Lean Mass Ratio (percent)—ratio of grip strength as determined by a hand dynamometer relative to amount of lean mass in the body

9. **Endurance**

Isometric Fatigue (seconds)—length of time the patient can perform an isometric exercise without stopping

Sit-Ups (number in sixty seconds)

Push-Ups (number)—with no time limit, but must be done without stopping

10. Vision

Static Visual Acuity (decimal)—ability of each eye to correctly discern letters at a given distance

Color Vision (number correct)—ability to discriminate numbers of a color embedded in a field of different colors

Pupillary Miosis (millimeters)—size of the pupil of the eye under normal lighting

11. Hearing

Pure Tone Threshold (db)—range of hearing the ear can discern for a tone, as opposed to speech

Speech Reception Threshold (db)—range of hearing of the ear to be able to detect speech

Once you have the test results available to you, you have established a base value for each test. This doesn't do a tremendous amount of good. What you really have is a single dot (for each test) on a separate graph. However, when you are tested the second time, you now have two dots on the graph and, not to oversimplify it, you connect the dots. When you have connected the dots, you have more than a straight line. You have a visual, quantifiable *trend*—both as to magnitude and direction. It tells you if you are growing younger or older and at what rate. It tells you how much you have become younger—or older—for each specific test, in terms of your biophysiological age. If you divide the sum total of all scores by the number of individual tests you took, it gives you the biophysiological age for your entire body.

Where do the scores—relative to age and gender—come from? Your physician should have them, or know where to get them. One of the reasons it took over two years to construct the L.I.F.E. TEST™ was that I created a database of more than *ten million* scores, stratified by gender and then by age, for each one of the forty-five different tests, measurements, and examinations. To my knowledge, it may still be the largest such database anywhere in the world. I consulted every known test of aging—the Baltimore Longitudinal Study of Aging, the Duke University Study, the Tucson Study, the studies from Tufts University, the Framingham studies, the National Disease and Therapeutic Index (NDTI), the National Health Interview Service (HIS), and others. I searched lab texts, clinical texts, professional journal articles, master's theses, and doctoral dissertations. I hounded government/private agencies/entities, such as NASA, the National Institute on Aging (NIA), the National Center for Health Statistics, the National Institutes of Health (NIH), and numerous other sources.

* * *

What I want you to do is look at the Appendices. If you are a woman, go to Appendix A; if you're a man, go to Appendix B. Look at the first score sheet, which will be for BODY COMPOSITION and, below it, PERCENT BODY FAT. Let's assume you are age 45, by the calendar. For the ladies, let's assume the sum of the five skinfold (the procedure to measure percent body fat) measurements is 64 mm. Look at the columns of figures. The first (leftmost number) is a chronological age. Then you see a dash, followed by two numbers separated by a slash. Find the number 64 to the right of a dash. You will see it located at age 35. What you see at that space is "35 - 64/24.7," which tells us that, if you have a skinfold total of 64 mm, it means that it is what a woman age 35 would have, and the percent body fat is 24.7. For the men, assume you have a skinfold total of 59 mm. If you locate 59 to the right of a dash, you see "43 - 59/22.6," which means you have the total of a man age 43, and the percent body fat is 22.6. For example, if a female, age 51, got a score of 47.8 years, this means she has the percent body fat of a female 47.8 years. If tested again at a later date (say, six months after the first test) and she got a score of 45.0 years, it means she now has the percent body fat of a female age 45.0 years *and* has become 2.8 years *younger* (as to percent body fat in that six-month period).

It is very important to be aware that, when you have located your score, the age at which that score appears becomes your biophysiological age—in this case, 35 for the ladies and 43 for the men. If you took the entire L.I.F.E. TEST™ you would have 45 different biological ages. Just add them all together and divide by 45. That gives you your overall, total, true biophysiological age. That's how old you *really* are.

I can't administer the L.I.F.E. TEST™ to you, and you can't administer it to yourself. Only your physician can administer the test and interpret the results. I also highly recommend that the physician be one who practices sports medicine or who has an exercise physiologist on staff. This will most likely insure the availability of the required equipment to administer the L.I.F.E. TEST™ and the knowledge to administer it. A good question would be whether or not you need to do all forty-five tests and whether you can substitute some from the list of biomarkers. The first answer is that you do not need to be administered all forty-five, but I would do at least thirty, *and at least one from each group*. The second answer is that you may, of course, substitute. You may well have a condition that prevents you from performing one or more tests. Only your physician is qualified to make that determination.

How much might this cost? When I had my National Center for Sports Medicine, the entire cost was $195. Was it covered by insurance? Not entirely. The extent of insurance coverage depends on what the insurance policy covers and the extent to which the tests would be appropriate to investigating the patient's symptoms. To give you an inside peek at health-care reimbursement, when you go to your physician for tests/treatment/procedures, he or she has a great big book of codes. Almost everything that can be done to you has a specific code. When the physician's insurance processor files the claim, the code number is put on the form. No code number, no reimbursement. In actual practice what I found was this: We could usually get about half the cost reimbursed by the insurance company, but it varied widely. The actual amount will vary by insurance policy and state.

*   *   *

What I have just given you is the method by which you can determine whether or not you are progressing, slowing down, or reversing the process of aging, depending on what you choose to do to your body. If you're wondering why I don't put the entire

L.I.F.E. TEST™ in this book, it is because the manual I created to explain the logic and process by which it was created, the equipment required to administer all the tests, the method used to actually administer each test (with pictures), and all the score sheets and the interpretations is over 400 pages in length.

*   *   *

It truly is irrelevant what claims advertisers make for their products' abilities to "make you younger." You can *prove* the veracity of the claim. The question is whether you want to spend the money to do it. And the claims are great in number and increasing. So, too, are the number of products that are involved. Perhaps the hottest "product" on the market today is human growth hormone (sometimes abbreviated as HGH or hGH, and also known as "humatrope"). If that looks familiar, it should. It is the same substance that I cite at the very beginning of chapter 6. HGH is just one group of hormones (DHEA, testosterone, pregnenolone, melatonin, estrogen, and progesterone are others) that are being used in a clinical setting for hormone replacement therapy (HRT).

The rise of HGH was stimulated several years ago by Daniel Rudman, M.D., and his colleagues at the Medical College of Wisconsin (Milwaukee). They administered controlled doses of HGH to twelve men, ages sixty-one to eighty-one, over a six-month period. The results were presented in an article in the *New England Journal of Medicine* (5 July 1990). The results of the study were impressive. The physiology of certain areas of the subjects' bodies had grown younger by *ten to twenty years*. Dr. Rudman followed this study with another one, with twenty-six elderly men. The results were good, though not as good as the previous study. Nonetheless, the theory that certain hormones decreased with age and, if administered in amounts to replace that which was lost, would have a "youthful, rejuvenating effect" on the patients was proven by classic, placebo-controlled, double-blind studies.

The administration of HGH is not without its dangers. In addition to acromegaly, there is some chance of the patient acquiring diabetes mellitus, to name two of the dangers. And HGH is not inexpensive. It could cost over $15,000 a year to receive the HRT utilizing HGH. The price has come down but still varies widely. It is manufactured by companies such as Genentech, Inc. and Eli Lilly and Company. The FDA has given its approval for HGH to be prescribed for HRT. Any reputable physician will tell you that you should *only* take HGH when administered by a licensed physician who monitors you for possible side effects. Unfortunately, the hucksters have gotten into the game and really wreaked havoc. What they are doing is offering HGH via the Internet, as well as through some "health/fitness" magazines. This is very dangerous. You do not know the purity of what you are getting. Some ads will add other substances, such as herbs, vitamins, and minerals, to make it seem to be "even more healthy" than HGH alone. Some manufacturers are selling a synthetic substance, which, while advertised as HGH, is *not* HGH. We simply don't know the possible side effects along with all the possible combinations of other substances, which may approach an infinite number.

*　*　*

Here are classic examples of how you get duped into buying "anti-aging" products. The potential sucker is around age forty. He or she is beginning to notice gray hairs, a spreading waistline, and what I call "gluteus spreaditis" (you know what it means). Perhaps the wrinkles are starting to show around the eyes and mouth. You can't seem to recover as quickly from a competitive sport contest. Your energy level seems to be less than only a few years before. You don't like wearing brightly colored clothes—they call too much attention to your once-beautiful body which is starting to go bad on you. The list seems to get longer every day.

Along comes somebody who claims to have the answer to all those problems. You think the ad seems reasonable enough. You have a little knowledge about the product being touted. You figure, "Why not? It can't hurt me." So you spend your money and . . . you have just been duped again. Over time, you keep repeating the process as you slowly become both more desperate and determined to solve this aging problem, especially if it seems so easy just to take some pills out of a bottle.

The ads for vitamins, minerals, herbs, ergogenic substances, and the like now substitute terms like "younger," "youth," and "antiaging" for terms like "vitamin insurance," "mineral balance," and "more muscle," and the list goes on and on. It is nothing but a variation on the same, tired, misleading, phony claims. But it works. And it will continue to work until you can prove or disprove the claims in your own situation.

This is a different slant than in all the previous chapters. Aging (or antiaging) didn't become big business until about five years ago. But the health and fitness industry found it could make billions just by changing the terms in its ads that had been used for the same products, but for different applications and a different audience.

There have been countless studies to disprove the claims in the areas covered in all earlier chapters in this book, but aging presents a new challenge. To truly prove or disprove a claim, you either have to do it on an individual basis (meaning you get your own test scores, which will cost you money), or you have to do a longitudinal study. A longitudinal study takes a lot of time and money. A longitudinal study requires that you take a group of people and follow them over a number of years and note changes as a result of taking or not taking some substance.

The longest-running, continuous longitudinal aging study is the Baltimore Longitudinal Study on Aging (BLSA). These types of studies are very difficult to do for a variety of reasons. The most obvious is that the subjects have to be available. We change residences quite often (on an average of once every five years). You have to keep all things in a person's life constant, save for one variable—the product or medicine you wish to administer over time to the group. Most people do not live constant lives, at least as far as their health and fitness is concerned. Of course, as people get older, they die, and they're obviously no longer part of the study. Many require prescription medications, which were not required when the study began, which can cause a "bias" in the study results—some new element has been introduced. Funding may be difficult to obtain, due to the exigencies coming out of Washington, D.C. Preliminary results of the study may be very discouraging and the study is halted. Something more important may take its place.

In a nutshell, if you want to do a longitudinal study on something like DHEA or HGH, it may take ten or more years. Do you think the hucksters are going to wait that long? So, the wheels of deceit are once again rolling on the highway to phony claims, a lack of concern for the customer, and a voracious hunger for quick profits.

To test my own intuition, I logged onto the Internet and typed in "human growth hormone" in the BellSouth default search engine. The number of "reviewed Web sites" displayed was 10,835. I tallied up the links on the first ten pages and found that 92 of the 100 Web sites were ads for people selling HGH or a "near substitute" (the seller's claim). And a significant number were from addresses (if one was given for the street/city/state/country address) from people in foreign countries, especially Canada.

Incredibly, some of the ads were from physicians—M.D.s—who were selling it through the mail. I did not verify if the people touting these degrees were, in fact, medical doctors.

You will also see a lot of ads for medical clinics where HGH is dispensed. The clinics are usually some sort of "antiaging" clinic. There's nothing wrong with that per se. What bothers me is that the claims made for HGH were, in many cases, unproven. I couldn't reproduce the ads because they are copyrighted and reproduction is not allowed. Somebody has good lawyers and/or is smart enough not to let them be reproduced and exposed in a book such as this.

I did pull one ad off the Internet that made me laugh. Look at the first two lines of the ad, below. Can anybody tell me what's wrong with it? It pushes wild blueberries as ". . . Nature's Anti-Aging Cure."[1] Follow me on this. The person who composed this headline has it exactly backward. If something is an antiaging cure, it means it *stops* something that *stops* aging. In effect it *facilitates* aging. The ad should have said it was a cure for aging, *not* a cure for *anti*aging. If you look at the rest of the ad, the mistake is repeated no less than two more times in a single paragraph. There has got to be some logical explanation why the noted Wild Blueberry Association of North America would say what it said. Isn't there some logical explanation? There is, isn't there? Well, I'm waiting . . .

*   *   *

Antioxidants From Wild Blueberries Are Nature's Anti-Aging Cure

If you are looking for information on any of the following topics:

- antioxidants
- antioxidant sources
- anti-aging cures
- anti-aging benefits

You'll find it at Wild Blueberry Association of North America!

Antioxidants are nature's anti-aging cure. Wild blueberries have been proven as one of the best antioxidant sources available in nature. With the complete nutrition that wild blueberries can provide, consumers can take advantage of anti-aging benefits by enjoying many of their favorite recipes. From blueberry pancakes to blueberry muffins, you'll never know that you're eating one of the best anti-aging cures available in stores today. Take advantage of nature's antioxidants today - enjoy the anti-aging benefits of wild blueberries today!

At Wild Blueberry Association of North America, you'll discover an easy to use, information-packed web site. Learn more about antioxidants.

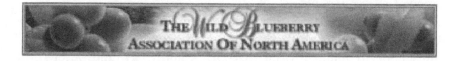

If you're wondering why I believe you can slow down the aging process and in some cases reverse it, let me explain. I believe you can do it, and measure the results as to magnitude and direction, as I have explained above. What I do *not* believe is that we are all going to live healthy, happy lives to age 130 or whatever the number is that is being bandied about by antiaging gurus. *I believe there is an absolute limit to how much you can slow down or reverse the aging process. It cannot continue forever. We are all going to die sooner or later. Some of the ads come so close to promising immortality, it's ludicrous.*

Because the body is so complex and its systems so intricately related, it does not seem possible that any single agent like DHEA or HGH can increase life span by an average of fifty years, which is exactly what proponents of these two hormones are saying.

The FDA banned nonprescription DHEA pills that claimed to help weight control. You have acquired enough knowledge from this book to know that supplements are not required to be proven safe or effective before they are marketed. That should tell you something.

As a student of genetics, I want to share something with you. Do you think that the reason DHEA and HGH levels fall as we get older is a defense mechanism; i.e., our bodies are not supposed to keep the same levels as we had when younger? Here's why I think it may be true. Some studies have shown that, when subjects were given DHEA and HGH (not at the same time), some subjects contracted certain cancers. This has also occurred in estrogen HRT. Is there something in these hormones that can trigger cancers in some people if levels exceed a certain amount at a given point in their lives? I don't know the answer. That's the problem. People got cancer, but we don't *know* whether or not it was due to HRT. It hasn't been proven that they *don't* cause cancer. For your health and safety, that bothers me—a lot.

All this fits into the same theme that has been touted before— beware of anybody who gives you only the "good" side of the story. I am willing to admit in print that DHEA and HGH (and other products) do have some proven benefits, but I also give you the downside. If you read the ads for these products, you almost never hear of cautions, dangers, or qualifiers. *That* is your best key that someone is either devious or ignorant (or both), but the intended result is the same—to convince you to spend your money.

Have you noticed something about the number of ads I have presented? The number has decreased as the book has progressed chapter by chapter. I did this for a specific reason. I wanted to wean you off the ads and replace it with knowledge. The more you read, the more you should be able to spot a phony ad. It serves no purpose to present the same theme over and over again, though the product may have changed.

There is nothing magical about spotting a phony ad. The more knowledge you acquire, the less likely you are to ever again have someone slap the label "SUCKER" on you.

I think it is time for me to stop tutoring you and to turn your life back over to you.

VIPS

Aging is a progressive process that can be slowed down, or reversed, but only to some finite limit.

You measure age, and the rate of change in aging, by measuring biomarkers of aging.

The body is too complex and its systems too intricately interrelated to be able to reverse the aging process by one single agent, whether it's a pill, a potion, or a hormone.

The biggest change—beneficial or detrimental—to your body will occur at the very beginning of any program or intervention.

Your greatest weaknesses that will allow you to become a sucker for any antiaging scheme are your ignorance, your ego, your desperation, your frustrations, and your unwillingness to believe that the next promised "cure" can't be another scam.

The last chapter is short, crisp, and concise. It is a summary, the culmination of the knowledge and tactics I have presented in this book for the benefit of your health and safety.

If you follow its checklists, you will never be duped again.

NOTE

1. The Wild Blueberry Association of North America ad, taken from Internet address: http://www.wildblueberries.com/antioxidants_hot.html [31 October 1999], p. 1 of 1.

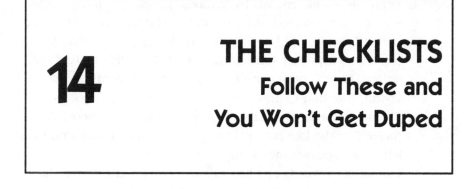

THE CHECKLISTS
Follow These and You Won't Get Duped

14

These checklists will be brief. If a checklist is too brief, it invites errors of omissions to critical items. If it is too long, it becomes so unwieldy as to be an impediment, rather than an aid, to the user. The entire objective of these checklists is to keep you from ever being duped again.

"DO NOT BUY" CHECKLIST

Do *not* purchase any health and fitness product or service if any of the following applies.

1. The ad contains any adjectives such as "unbelievable," "revolutionary," "astounding," and the like.
2. The product or service can't or hasn't been proven by the scientific method.
3. The seller says it has been "scientifically proven." Ask for the journal title and issue in which the product or service was written up, and then go look it up for yourself. Only accept the scientific evidence if it has been shown to apply to the population in general, not just a few subjects in the study.

4. There are endorsements by "famous" people, or testimonials.

5. Any results claimed do not state whether or not those claimed results can be expected by the majority of users.

6. The claim says that something "might" help this or that condition. It will or it won't. "Might" is just another way of saying, "We don't know if it will or it won't."

7. The ad contains nonquantitative claims such as "more," "less," "better," or the like rather than specific, quantifiable amounts within a specific time period.

8. The ad uses words or phrases such as "all natural" that have no accepted meaning in the scientific community.

9. The ad states that vitamins, minerals, or other supplements provide energy, or replace those that have been "robbed" from your body, or have other exorbitant claims attached to them.

10. The ad makes a diagnosis for a condition that only your physician, after taking a medical history, performing necessary tests, and interpreting the specific results could recommend that you take any particular drug and/or supplement.

11. The ad is from a source you don't know and trust.

12. The product is sold through a multilevel marketing company.

13. The ad contains some "health questionnaire" that you fill out to determine if you need to buy the product.

14. The product was made in the People's Republic of China.

15. You don't know the meaning of *all* the ingredients.

16. The ad is for any type of exercise equipment that does not allow for a full ROM (Range Of Motion), and does not state that it's the FID (Frequency, Intensity, and Duration) that makes it effective, not some "revolutionary, technical advancement."

17. You don't know the meaning of, don't recognize, or can't verify someone's credentials (with respect to a license, certification, or registration).

18. The advice comes from a "professional" advisor who has financial interest in any product he or she recommends to you.

19. The ad is for any weight-loss program. Remember, the odds are twenty-to-one *against* you being successful in attaining a permanent weight loss.

20. The ad is for some antiaging product, unless you have your physician's approval in advance.
21. Don't let your ego, emotions, or desperation make you a sucker.

THE "DO" CHECKLIST

This checklist includes things you can do, irrespective and apart from, any ads that you encounter.

1. Read this book and refer to it often.
2. Buy free weights if you want the least expensive, longest-lasting, and most effective resistance "equipment" ever made.
3. Provide as much information about yourself as possible when you go to your personal physician for advicc. This should include—at minimum—your name, age, gender, and specific goal(s); any ads or information that relates to what it is you are seeking advice about; a specific list of every prescription and nonprescription drug or supplement you are currently taking or have taken in the last thirty days; the list you should absolutely create (see #7, below); any specific health/fitness complaints or problems you have; and what specific advice/ service(s) you wish your physician to perform.
4. Subscribe to the *free* health/fitness reports I listed in chapter 10.
5. Read the information on http://www.ncahf.org and http:// www.quackwatch.com.
6. Have at least an annual test for your levels of iron (especially for women) and any other levels of vitamins and minerals you believe you may be lacking in adequate amounts.
7. Make a list of everything you eat and drink for thirty days; get one of the recommended books on nutrition listed in the bibliography; and compute (please, do this just once in your life—for your own health) the amounts of vitamins, minerals, fat, protein, and carbohydrates that you consume on an *average daily basis*. Take this with you when you see your personal physician.

8. Visit your physician or other trusted health and fitness advisor in his or her office.

9. Deliberately look at, and listen to, ads for health and fitness products. Try and see what is wrong with the ads. It won't take long.

10. Support any proconsumer legislation, especially anything that will put the burden of proof for claims on the seller, and would require manufacturers and sellers to prove their claims *before* their products are offered for sale.

<table>
<tr><td>

APPENDIX A

</td><td>

WOMEN'S BIOMARKERS OF AGING
Female L.I.F.E. Test™
Score Sheets
(Refer to pages 293–94)

</td></tr>
</table>

FEMALE

TEST GROUP: BODY COMPOSITION
TEST TYPE: PERCENT BODY FAT
SUBTEST TYPE/TYPE OF MEASUREMENT (IF ANY):
   SUM OF 5 SKINFOLDS
UNIT(S) OF MEASURE: MILLIMETERS (mm)
MEASURING EQUIPMENT USED: SKINFOLD CALIPER

AGE—SCORES

21—54/21.3	35—64/24.7	49—83/30.0	63—93/33.9
22—54/21.4	36—66/25.0	50—84/30.1	64—93/34.2
23—55/21.5	37—67/25.3	51—85/30.4	65—93/34.3
24—56/21.8	38—71/25.8	52—86/30.8	66—94/34.9
25—56/22.0	39—72/26.1	53—87/31.1	67—95/35.3
26—57/22.2	40—73/26.4	54—88/31.3	68—95/35.6
27—58/22.3	41—75/27.1	55—89/31.6	69—96/35.9
28—59/22.5	42—76/27.2	56—89/31.8	70—96/36.1
29—59/22.6	43—77/27.8	57—90/32.0	71—97/36.5
30—60/22.7	44—78/28.4	58—90/32.3	72—97/36.9
31—62/23.0	45—79/28.6	59—91/32.6	73—98/37.3
32—63/23.4	46—80/28.8	60—91/32.8	74—98/37.8
33—63/24.0	47—82/29.5	61—92/33.3	75—99/38.0
34—63/24.4	48—83/29.9	62—92/33.5	

FEMALE

TEST GROUP: PULMONARY RESPIRATORY
TEST TYPE: FORCED VITAL CAPACITY (FVC)
SUBTEST TYPE/TYPE OF MEASUREMENT (IF ANY):
> 68" HEIGHT
UNIT(S) OF MEASURE: MILLILITERS (ml)
MEASURING EQUIPMENT USED: SPIROMETER

AGE—SCORES

21—4328	35—3938	49—3726	63—3489
22—4209	36—3908	50—3709	64—3480
23—4174	37—3888	51—3685	65—3473
24—4157	38—3869	52—3663	66—3468
25—4140	39—3855	53—3651	67—3462
26—4116	40—3840	54—3629	68—3458
27—4092	41—3821	55—3615	69—3456
28—4078	42—3802	56—3605	70—3454
29—4063	43—3790	57—3585	71—3427
30—4049	44—3785	58—3570	72—3412
31—4022	45—3771	59—3557	73—3389
32—4000	46—3758	60—3544	74—3374
33—3974	47—3750	61—3520	75—3368
34—3956	48—3740	62—3500	

FEMALE

TEST GROUP: PULMONARY RESPIRATORY
TEST TYPE: FORCED VITAL CAPACITY (FVC)
SUBTEST TYPE/TYPE OF MEASUREMENT (IF ANY):
   62-68" HEIGHT
UNIT(S) OF MEASURE: MILLILITERS (ml)
MEASURING EQUIPMENT USED: SPIROMETER

AGE—SCORES

21—3938	35—3675	49—3419	63—3187
22—3912	36—3655	50—3408	64—3170
23—3886	37—3634	51—3397	65—3160
24—3867	38—3617	52—3384	66—3151
25—3852	39—3597	53—3365	67—3130
26—3827	40—3578	54—3355	68—3111
27—3817	41—3555	55—3327	69—3099
28—3804	42—3530	56—3308	70—3082
29—3793	43—3513	57—3281	71—3062
30—3781	44—3497	58—3262	72—3043
31—3752	45—3482	59—3250	73—3043
32—3726	46—3461	60—3232	74—3022
33—3707	47—3450	61—3215	75—3017
34—3695	48—3438	62—3202	

FEMALE

TEST GROUP: PULMONARY RESPIRATORY
TEST TYPE: FORCED VITAL CAPACITY (FVC)
SUBTEST TYPE/TYPE OF MEASUREMENT (IF ANY):
    < 62" HEIGHT
UNIT(S) OF MEASURE: MILLILITERS (ml)
MEASURING EQUIPMENT USED: SPIROMETER

AGE—SCORES

21—3636	35—3399	49—3168	63—2883
22—3621	36—3378	50—3153	64—2871
23—3604	37—3362	51—3130	65—2865
24—3586	38—3351	52—3101	66—2851
25—3570	39—3342	53—3080	67—2843
26—3551	40—3315	54—3059	68—2836
27—3532	41—3298	55—3038	69—2827
28—3515	42—3283	56—3017	70—2819
29—3504	43—3272	57—2996	71—2801
30—3489	44—3251	58—2980	72—2776
31—3471	45—3230	59—2961	73—2763
32—3459	46—3218	60—2947	74—2747
33—3432	47—3205	61—2924	75—2733
34—3419	48—3182	62—2901	

FEMALE

TEST GROUP: CORONARY HEART DISEASE
TEST TYPE: SERUM TOTAL CHOLESTEROL
SUBTEST TYPE/TYPE OF MEASUREMENT (IF ANY):
UNIT(S) OF MEASURE: MIILIGAMS PER DECALITER (mg/dl)
MEASURING EQUIPMENT USED: BLOOD DRAWING TRAY,
     CORVAC VIAL

AGE—SCORES

21—178	35—191	49—220	63—239
22—179	36—193	50—222	64—240
23—180	37—194	51—223	65—242
24—182	38—196	52—225	66—243
25—183	39—198	53—227	67—246
26—184	40—200	54—229	68—244
27—185	41—201	55—230	69—242
28—185	42—203	56—231	70—241
29—186	43—205	57—232	71—239
30—186	44—207	58—233	72—236
31—187	45—210	59—234	73—232
32—188	46—212	60—235	74—230
33—189	47—216	61—236	75—229
34—190	48—218	62—237	

MEN'S BIOMARKERS OF AGING
Male L.I.F.E. Test™
Score Sheets

(Refer to pages 293–94)

MALE

TEST GROUP: BODY COMPOSITION
TEST TYPE: PERCENT BODY FAT
SUBTEST TYPE/TYPE OF MEASUREMENT (IF ANY):
    SUM OF 5 SKINFOLDS
UNIT(S) OF MEASURE: MILLIMETERS (mm)
MEASURING EQUIPMENT USED: SKINFOLD CALIPER

AGE—SCORES

21—44/19.8	35—55/21.6	49—63/23.3	63—64/24.7
22—45/19.9	36—55/21.7	50—63/23.4	64—64/24.8
23—46/20.0	37—55/21.7	51—64/23.5	65—64/24.9
24—47/20.0	38—56/21.9	52—64/23.6	66—65/24.9
25—48/20.1	39—56/22.0	53—64/23.6	67—65/24.8
26—49/20.2	40—57/22.1	54—63/23.7	68—66.24.7
27—50.20.4	41—57/22.2	55—63/23.8	69—66/24.6
28—50/20.6	42—58/22.4	56—63/23.9	70—66/24.5
29—51/20.7	43—59/22.6	57—63/24.0	71—67/24.4
30—52/20.8	44—60/22.7	58—63/24.1	72—67/24.3
31—52/20.9	45—61/22.8	59—63/24.2	73—67/24.2
32—53/21.0	46—62/22.9	60—63/24.4	74—67/24.1
33—54/21.2	47—62/23.0	61—64/24.5	75—67/24.0
34—54/21.4	48—62/23.2	62—64/24.6	

MALE

TEST GROUP: PULMONARY RESPIRATORY
TEST TYPE: FORCED VITAL CAPACITY (FVC)
SUBTEST TYPE/TYPE OF MEASUREMENT (IF ANY):
> 74" HEIGHT
UNIT(S) OF MEASURE: MILLILITERS (ml)
MEASURING EQUIPMENT USED: SPIROMETER

AGE—SCORES

21—5650	35—5245	49—4958	63—4663
22—5620	36—5206	50—4945	64—4640
23—5580	37—5168	51—4916	65—4630
24—5560	38—5151	52—4876	66—4621
25—5520	39—5142	53—4852	67—4616
26—5470	40—5130	54—4833	68—4609
27—5450	41—5107	55—4820	69—4605
28—5430	42—5082	56—4772	70—4605
29—5415	43—5062	57—4755	71—4582
30—5398	44—5051	58—4748	72—4553
31—5361	45—5042	59—4735	73—4526
32—5337	46—5030	60—4702	74—4507
33—5304	47—5017	61—4693	75—4490
34—5261	48—4973	62—4671	

MALE

TEST GROUP: PULMONARY RESPIRATORY
TEST TYPE: FORCED VITAL CAPACITY (FVC)
SUBTEST TYPE/TYPE OF MEASUREMENT (IF ANY):
    68-74" HEIGHT
UNIT(S) OF MEASURE: MILLILITERS (ml)
MEASURING EQUIPMENT USED: SPIROMETER

AGE—SCORES

21—5251	35—4900	49—4574	63—4246
22—5228	36—4876	50—4563	64—4238
23—5184	37—4837	51—4540	65—4230
24—5161	38—4803	52—4512	66—4201
25—5136	39—4796	53—4473	67—4176
26—5102	40—4782	54—4439	68—4151
27—5086	41—4741	55—4422	69—4127
28—5068	42—4720	56—4402	70—4109
29—5055	43—4684	57—4375	71—4080
30—5042	44—4664	58—4350	72—4062
31—5011	45—4640	59—4329	73—4051
32—4973	46—4616	60—4310	74—4037
33—4953	47—4600	61—4286	75—4022
34—4927	48—4584	62—4262	

MALE

TEST GROUP: PULMONARY RESPIRATORY
TEST TYPE: FORCED VITAL CAPACITY (FVC)
SUBTEST TYPE/TYPE OF MEASUREMENT (IF ANY):
    < 68" HEIGHT
UNIT(S) OF MEASURE: MILLILITERS (ml)
MEASURING EQUIPMENT USED: SPIROMETER

AGE—SCORES

21—4848	35—4527	49—4218	63—3855
22—4818	36—4507	50—4917	64—3835
23—4800	37—4482	51—4168	65—3820
24—4781	38—4468	52—4134	66—3801
25—4730	39—4459	53—4120	67—3784
26—4730	40—4448	54—4070	68—3772
27—4701	41—4412	55—4048	69—3764
28—4681	42—4380	56—4017	70—3758
29—4670	43—4362	57—3994	71—3724
30—4652	44—4339	58—3953	72—3696
31—4631	45—4325	59—3929	73—3671
32—4604	46—4304	60—3910	74—3659
33—4572	47—4271	61—3899	75—3644
34—4558	48—4243	62—3872	

MALE

TEST GROUP: CORONARY HEART DISEASE
TEST TYPE: SERUM TOTAL CHOLESTEROL
SUBTEST TYPE/TYPE OF MEASUREMENT (IF ANY):
UNIT(S) OF MEASURE: MIILIGAMS PER DECALITER (mg/dl)
MEASURING EQUIPMENT USED: BLOOD DRAWING TRAY,
    CORVAC VIAL

AGE—SCORES

21—175	35—207	49—225	63—234
22—177	36—208	50—228	64—235
23—180	37—210	51—228	65—235
24—182	38—211	52—229	66—234
25—184	39—212	53—229	67—233
26—187	40—213	54—230	68—232
27—190	41—214	55—230	69—232
28—193	42—217	56—230	70—232
29—195	43—218	57—231	71—232
30—197	44—219	58—231	72—231
31—199	45—221	59—232	73—229
32—201	46—222	60—232	74—227
33—203	47—223	61—232	75—225
34—205	48—224	62—233	

GLOSSARY

Absorption. The process of intake of liquids by solids, or of gases by liquids or solids. As it relates to digestion, it is the passage of some substance through the body's surfaces into body fluids and tissues and changed into other substances to be utilized by the body or passed out the end of the digestive system as waste.

Adequate Intake (AI). The amount of vitamins and minerals that is sufficient for more than 98 percent of all normally healthy adults.

ADP (adenosine diphosphate). A compound of adenosine containing two phosphoric acid groups. It is produced during muscle contraction. It is reformed when the muscle relaxes.

Adrenalin. The British designation for epinephrine.

Aging. A progression of changes at the cellular level, caused by internal and external forces, which will eventually result in the death of the organism.

Aldosterone. A hormone produced by the adrenal cortex that regulates sodium ion reabsorption.

"All natural." No definition. This is a phrase created by the hucksters in the health and fitness industry for marketing purposes to sell their products.

Anabolism. The constructive or growth phase of metabolism. It is often used with the word "steroid"—as in "anabolic steroid"—to denote a class of drugs used by athletes to increase size and strength.

Androgens. Substances producing or stimulating the development of male characteristics (masculinization), such as the hormones testosterone and androsterone.

Anorexia. Loss of appetite or desire for food.

Antioxidants. An agent that prevents oxidation (the process of a substance combining with oxygen). It is theorized that certain nutrients—especially vitamins A, C, and E—may possibly play a role in the prevention of certain cancers by destroying free radicals. Free radicals are molecules containing an odd number of electrons that contain an open bond or a half bond and are highly reactive. There has been no conclusive scientific evidence as to the cause-and-effect of antioxidants and cancer prevention.

Antioxidation. The prevention or inhibition of the process of substances combining with oxygen.

"Approved." No definition. It is usually employed by industry hucksters to imply some sort of "official and legitimate" approval or recommendation when, in fact, no such official and legitimate approval exists.

ATP (adenosine triphosphate). An organic molecule that stores and releases chemical energy for use in body cells.

Basal metabolic rate (BMR). The amount of energy expended by the body when in a resting state. It is the most important factor in the determination of weight gain or loss.

Beta-carotene (also ß-carotene). The precursor to vitamin A.

Bicarbonate buffer system. The interaction of bicarbonate and agents in the blood that tend to offset the reaction of an agent in conjunction with the bicarbonate.

Biomarkers of aging. A functional part of the human body which can be physiologically tested, measured, and examined to determine the age-associated characteristics of the organ or system. It is a number that represents the result of the test, measurement, or examination.

Biophysiological age. The *true* age of an organism. It is not the chronological (calendar) age. It is the sum total of the major organs' and systems' physiological state at a point in time.

Body Mass Index (BMI). The ratio of weight (in kilograms) divided by height (in meters squared). The result is body composition; i.e., the degree of fat in the body.

Brain (energy metabolism). The sum total of all the chemical reactions that take place in all the cells within the brain.

Cadmium. A metallic element whose salts are poisonous.

Calcitonin. A hormone released by the thyroid that promotes a decrease in the level of calcium in the blood.

Carbohydrates. A group of chemical substances, including glycogen, starches, sugars, dextrins, and celluloses, that contain only carbon, oxygen, and hydrogen. The ratio of hydrogen to oxygen is usually 2:1.

Catabolism. The destructive phase of metabolism. The opposite of anabolism.

Caveat emptor. A Latin phrase meaning "Let the buyer beware."

Caveat vendor. A Latin phrase meaning "Let the seller beware."

Cellulite. A nontechnical term for the deposits of fat at the subcutaneous level, especially in the thighs, legs, and buttocks. It is not a different or unusual type of fat. It is like any other body fat, but hucksters use the word to sell weight loss and anticellulite products, all of which are worthless.

Chelation therapy. A series of intravenous infusions containing disodium edatate and various other substances.

Chromium. An essential trace element required by the body for normal glucose metabolism.

"Clinically proven." No definition. Used by hucksters to add a phony layer of respectability and acceptability to their products. It is usually found that the clinic does not exist (if stated), is not a legitimate clinic, or is only part of many larger studies and taken out of context to "prove" how wonderful a product is.

Coenzyme Q-10 (also called ubiquinol). The reduced form of coenzyme Q, present in virtually all cells, and is a collector of reducing equivalents during intracellular respiration.

Collagen. A fibrous, insoluble protein found in the connective tissue, including skin, bones, ligaments, and cartilage.

Complex carbohydrates. Dietary starch.

Control group. Subjects used in a study that are given a placebo and not the real agent being studied.

Corticosteroids. Steroid hormones released by the adrenal cortex.

Creatinine. The creatine anhydrid, which is a normal metabolic waste.

Daily Reference Values (DRV). DRVs are used for macronutrients—fat, carbohydrates, protein, fiber, sodium, and potassium—and are based upon a diet containing 60 percent carbohydrate, 10 percent protein, 30 percent fat (including 10 percent saturated fat), and 11.5 grams of fiber per 1,000 calories.

Daily Value (DV). Daily Values combine the information from two sets of reference values—the Reference Dietary Intakes (RDIs) and Daily Reference Values (DRVs), neither of which appears on the labels themselves. The Daily Values are based on daily diets of 2,000 and 2,500 calories (the label will state which amount of calories the Daily Values are based upon). Individuals are advised to adjust the values to correspond with their own caloric intake.

Dehydroepiandrosterone (DHEA). A hormone and an androgenic (causing muscularization) substance, present in the urine.

Dermatitis. An inflammation of the skin.

Dietary Reference Intake (DRI). DRI encompasses four other categories of values: Estimated Average Requirement (EAR), Recommended Dietary Allowance (RDA), Adequate Intake (AI), and Tolerable Upper Intake Level (UL). DRIs do *not* include DV, DRI, RDI, or USDRA.

Dimethyl sulfoxide (DMSO). A solvent used to facilitate the absorption of medicines through the skin.

Dopamine receptors. The components of cells that act to attract and attach dopamine to those cells.

Double-blind. A technique used in the method of scientific investigation wherein neither the subject(s) nor the investigator(s) working with the subject(s) know what treatment, if any, the subject(s) is receiving. This technique is used to eliminate bias in the observer and the subject.

Dysphagia. The inability to swallow or difficulty in swallowing.

Elastin. The main protein in the elastic fibers of connective tissues.

Endopeptidase. A proteolytic enzyme that cleaves peptides in their centers more than at their ends.

Energy. The capacity of an organism or system to do work. Changes in energy can be physical, chemical, or both.

Enzyme. A protein that acts as a biological catalyst to speed up the body's metabolism (chemical reactions).

Epinephrine (adrenalin). The chief hormone produced by the adrenal medulla.

Ergogenic aids. Substances (supplements), usually in pill, powder, or liquid form, taken for the purpose of increasing potential for work output (energy).

Estimated Average Requirement (EAR). The estimated nutrient need of 50 percent of the individuals within any specific group.

Estradiol. A steroid produced by the ovary and possessing estrogenic (feminization) properties.

Estrogen. The female sex hormones, specifically estradiol and estrone.

Experimental group. Subjects in a study that are given the real agent, not the placebo.

Extracellular fluids. Fluids which lie outside the cells of the body. This includes plasma and interstitial fluid.

Fat. Adipose tissue in the body, which is used as a store of energy.

"Fat free." A misleading term. It does not mean a food or drink is entirely free of fat. A food or drink is considered "fat free" if it contains less than 0.5 grams per serving (not container).

FDA. Food and Drug Administration. The official U.S. regulatory body for cosmetics, drugs, foods, and medical devices. It is part of the Department of Health and Human Services.

Ferritin. An iron-phosphorous-protein complex containing about 23 percent iron. Ferritin is the form in which iron is stored in the tissues, primarily of the spleen, liver, and bone marrow.

FEV_1 (forced expiratory volume). Amount of air that can be forcefully exhaled from the lungs in one second.

Folic acid. A member of the vitamin B complex. Found naturally in green plant tissue, liver, and yeast.

FVC (forced vital capacity). Amount of air that can be exhaled from the lungs after the individual breathes in as deeply as possible. There is no time limit for FVC, but the exhalation must be continuous until no more air can be expelled.

Genes. The basic heredity unit, and is a microscopic, self-producing structure which is capable of creating a new like-kind structure or, if mutated incorrectly, producing a nonlike-kind structure. Hereditary traits are controlled by pairs of genes, called "alleles," located in the same position on a pair of chromosomes.

Globulin. One of a group of simple proteins insoluble in pure water but soluble in neutral solutions of salts of strong acids. When in the serum of the blood, it is the fraction of blood serum with which antibodies are associated.

Glucose. The principal blood sugar.

Glutathione. A tripeptide of glutamic acid, cysteine, and glycine, which takes up and gives of oxygen and is fundamentally important in cellular respiration.

Glycogenesis. The breakdown of glycogen to glucose.

Glycolisis. Breakdown of glucose to pyruvic acid—an anaerobic process.

Goiter. An enlargement of the thyroid gland.

Gout. Hereditary metabolic disease that is a form of acute arthritis and is marked by inflammation of the joints.

Hematocrit. The percentage of erythrocytes (red blood cells) to total blood volume.

Hemoglobin. The oxygen-transporting components of red blood cells.

Hemolytic anemia. Reduction of oxygen due to reduction of oxygen-carrying ability of red blood cells due to their rupture.

Herbs. Plants with soft stems that contain little, if any, wood. The term is used in health and fitness to denote a plant that supposedly possesses some medicinal value.

Homeopathy. A pseudoscience based on the notion that (a) a substance that produces symptoms in a healthy person can cure ill people with similar symptoms, and (b) that infinitesimal doses can be highly potent.

Ions. Atoms with either a positive or negative electrical charge.

Kilocalories. A unit of measure for heat. When it is used in nutrition, it is written as a capital "C."

Lipids. Any of a group of fats or fatlike substances, characterized by their insolubility in water, and solubility in fat solvents such as alcohol, ether, and chloroform.

Lipoproteins. Paired proteins consisting of simple proteins combined with lipid components: cholesterol, phospholipid, and triglyceride. Lipoproteins are classified as VLDL—very-low-density lipoproteins; LDL—low-density lipoproteins; and HDL—high-density lipoproteins. The density refers to the amount of protein to lipids.

"Little League elbow." A form of overuse syndrome in which there is an inflammation of the medial condyle of the elbow.

Lymphoma. Any of the various, abnormally proliferative diseases of the lymph gland or the lymphatic system.

M-1 and M-2. Names given to genes that appear to have some capability to control the life span of a human. It has not been proven conclusively that these are truly "immortality" genes, or even that any do exist.

Melanin. Dark pigment formed by cells' melanocytes; imparts color to the skin and hair.

Melatonin. Hormone produced by the pineal gland (in the brain).

Membrane permeability. The ability to allow substances to enter and exit a cell through the outer skin (membrane) of the cell.

Metabolic Equivalent (MET). A relative measure of energy expenditure. One MET is equivalent to the expenditure of the body while at rest. All other activities are considered multiples of this resting state. For example, if an activity is said to be 8 METs, that activity results in eight times the energy expended by the body while at rest.

Metabolism. Physical and chemical changes that take place within an organism. When correctly used, it is used with a qualifying word, such as "fat metabolism," "Carbohydrate metabolism," and "carbohydrate metabolism." When applied to the sum total of all the metabolisms within an organism, it is called the "organism's metabolism." It is often incorrectly used by hucksters when they say something like, "It will increase your metabolism" and you (and usually the hucksters) have no idea whether they are referring to one kind of metabolism or the organism's metabolism.

Minerals. Inorganic (possessing no carbon atoms) compounds or elements occurring in nature, most often in a solid state.

Minimum Daily Requirement (MDR). The amount of nutrients below which, if a person consumed that lower amount, that person would likely suffer various maladies due to a nutritional deficiency.

Multilevel marketing (MLM). A business organization constructed with an ever-larger number of sales representatives as the pyramid descends to lower and lower levels. They are most often used to employ individuals to push products that are used frequently, such as phone service, health and fitness products, cosmetics, and the like. Usually, very little formal training is given to the sales reps, who are almost always not employees, but independent contractors, and very seldom make any money for their efforts.

"Natural." Not abnormal or artificial. Often used with the word "all"—as in "all natural." It is used by hucksters to make consumers believe something is just as it exists in nature, without human intervention, and that is almost always a lie. Especially used when referring to vitamins, minerals, and herbs which are synthesized (artificially produced in a lab), but touted as being "natural," when that is exactly what they are *not*.

Neuritis. Inflammation of the nerves.

Neurotransmitters. Chemicals released by neurons that may, upon binding to receptors of neurons or effector cells, stimulate or inhibit them.

Neutrophils. The most abundant type of white blood cells.

Noradrenaline (norepinephrine). A hormone produced by the adrenal medulla, similar in chemical and pharmacological properties to epinephrine, but chiefly a constrictor of blood vessels with little effect on cardiac output.

Nucleic acids. A group of high molecular weight substances—such as DNA—found in cells of all living things.

Nutrition. The sum total of all the processes of ingesting and utilizing food and liquids by which growth, maintenance, and repair of activities of the body as a whole or any of its parts is accomplished.

Obesity. A state of being at least 30 percent above a person's individual ideal weight.

Office of Alternative Medicine (OAM). Renamed the National Center for Complementary and Alternative Medicine (NCCAM), it is a component of the National Institutes of Health, and was established to stimulate research into "alternative methods." So far, NCCAM and its predecessors have sponsored very little meaningful research, have never criticized anything as ineffective, and have tended to refer people seeking more information to unreliable sources. To date, none of the sponsored research has demonstrated that anything studied is effective.

Organic. Pertaining to carbon-containing substances, such as proteins, fats, and carbohydrates.

Osmotic pressure. Water-attracting ability of plasma proteins.

Osteomalacia. A disease marked by the increased softening of the bones, so that they become flexible and brittle, thus causing deformities. The adult form of osteomalacia is called rickets.

Osteoporosis. Increased softening of the bone resulting in a gradual decrease in the rate of bone formation.

Parathyroid hormones (PTH). Hormone released by the thyroid glands that regulates blood calcium levels.

Pellagra. A deficiency disease or syndrome endemic to certain parts of the world, characterized by cutaneous, gastrointestinal, neurologic, and mental symptoms.

Peptides. A class of substances prepared by synthesis of amino acids and intermediate in molecular weight and chemical properties between the amino acids, which can be made artificially, and the proteins, which cannot.

PH balance. The relative proportion of acidity or alkalinity of a substance; pH stands for potential of hydrogen. The neutral point, where a substance is neither acidic or alkaline is 7. Increasing acidity is expressed in a number less than 7; increasing alkalinity is expressed in a number greater than 7. Maximum acidity is 0 (zero) and maximum alkalinity is 14. The numbers are in a logarithm scale, and each whole number is a tenfold difference to the next highest or lowest number to that number.

Placebo. A totally inactive substance. It is usually given to a control group in a scientific study so that neither the control group nor the experimental group (which is given the active, real substance) knows which substance is the "real" one and which one is not. A placebo should look, taste, feel, and smell just like the real substance.

Power output. The amount of kinetic energy generated by the entire body in motion.

Precursor. A substance that precedes another substance, sometimes in the manufacture or creation of the following substance.

Progesterone. Hormone responsible for preparing the uterus for the fertilized ovum.

Prostatic specific antigen (PSA). A protein marker on the surface of the cells in the blood that may indicate cancer of the prostate.

Proteins. Complex nitrogenous substances; the main building material of cells.

Proteolytic. A process which hastens a reaction in proteins in which water is one of the reactants.

Puffery. Statements allowed by law that are not considered to be decisive factors in a decision to purchase an item. The general public is assumed to know that "puffed" statements may be false, but are not relying on them as true in making the decision to purchase or not purchase an item. The line between puffery and fraud is often indistinguishable. Hucksters often cross this line with impunity.

Pyramiding. A marketing scheme where only the individuals at the top of the "pyramid" can ever hope to make any money. Most pyramid schemes are blatantly illegal, and are solely designed to attract ever-increasing amounts of money from investors at lower levels, until such time as the scam artists decide to simply "take the money and run."

Reaction speed. The length of time it takes the body to respond to a visual stimulation resulting in a movement of the appropriate part, or parts, of the body.

Recommended Dietary Allowance (RDA). The amount of nutrients that are perfectly adequate for 97 to 98 percent of all healthy adults in America. It is an amount which need not be exceeded to insure adequate intake.

Reference Daily Intake (RDI). The amount of nutrients based on the 1968 National Academy of Sciences research and computations of the then-current RDA. The RDI are for twelve vitamins and seven minerals based on the 1968 RDAs.

Rickets. The adult form of osteomalacia.

Sawtooth palmetto. An herb that contains plant sterols that improve physical performance, and has profound effects on testosterone metabolism.

Sciatica. Severe pain in the leg along the course of the sciatic nerve, felt at the back of the thigh and running down the inside of the leg.

Scientific method. A specific set of procedures used to prove or disprove whether something can be proven true or not. It often attempts to prove whether or not a cause-and-effect situation exists. It can have several distinct steps but, when involving human beings, will always require selection of a control and experimental group, be placebo-controlled, be double-blind, and results will be reported with absolute truth and without bias to one or more legitimate scientific journals for publication. A correctly designed scientific study should be able to be reproduced (replicated) by anybody, and show the same results.

Scientifically proven. When used correctly, it means that the effect of the use of some has been shown to exist in studies employing only the scientific method. When used incorrectly, most often by hucksters, it can mean *anything* the huckster wants it to mean, but *not* that it was proven by the scientific method.

Scurvy. A deficiency disease characterized by hemorrhagic manifestations and abnormal functions of bone and teeth.

Selenium. A chemical element resembling sulfur. It is a trace mineral, functions as an antioxidant, and complements the role of vitamin E function.

Serotonin. A neurotransmitter of the central nervous system, often associated with sleep and fatiguing conditions.

Somatomedin (A and C). A group of insulin-like growth factors that require growth hormone in order to exert their function of stimulating growth.

Somatostatin. A hormone that inhibits the release of somatotropin, another growth hormone.

Steroid hormones. The sex hormones and the hormones of the adrenal cortex.

Sterols. One of a group of substances related to fats and belonging to the lipids. An example is cholesterol.

Stratification. The process of separating or differentiating one or more groups from all other groups in that universe.

Stromelysin. An extracellular endopeptidase of various tissues.

Submax treadmill. The heart rate in beats per minute of exertion of a body on a treadmill in the first of three stages of difficulty (effort).

Superoxidase dismutase (DMSO). An enzyme in the body's first line of defense against antioxidants.

Synthetic vitamins. Vitamins produced in a laboratory. These are not vitamins taken from foods and plants that exist in a true natural state. Every vitamin—and supplement, for that matter—that is produced by anybody is a synthetic vitamin. Hucksters tout their products as "natural" or "all natural" but they are not. They are made in a lab.

Tachycardia. In general, an abnormally rapid heart rate exceeding one hundred beats per minute in adults. Some types of tachycardia, such as sinus tachycardia, are not abnormal; rather, these can be due to exercise, hyperthermia, and certain drugs such as nicotine, atropine, and epinephrine.

Thymus gland. An unpaired organ located in the mediastinal cavity in front of, and above, the heart.

Thymus hormones. Hormones produced and secreted by the thymus gland.

Trace minerals. Organic elements normally found in minute quantities in foods and tissues. Examples are aluminum, copper, iron, iodine, and chromium.

Triglycerides. Combination of glycerol with three of five different fatty acids, which are also called neutral fats. A large portion of the fatty substances, lipids, in the blood is triglycerides.

"Undernourished." No definition accepted in medicine or science. It is often confused with the word "undernutrition"—as explained below—to denote the state of lacking in one or some (but usually several) key dietary nutrients.

Undernutrition. Inadequate nutrition from any cause.

Upper Intake Level (UL). This is the "Do not exceed" level of nutrient intake. If this level is exceeded, there is a 50/50 chance of suffering some toxic effects from that of those excess or excesses.

U.S. Recommended Daily Allowance (USRDA). A simplified FDA version of the 1968 RDAs that was used for many years in food labeling. It has been replaced by RDIs.

Vitamins. Any group of organic (possessing carbon atoms) substances *other* than minerals, proteins, carbohydrates, fats, or organic salts, essential for the normal growth, metabolism, and development of the human body. They are, most simply, chemicals bound together. They provide no energy whatsoever.

VO_2 Max. Maximum uptake of oxygen by the body.

Wellness. No definition. This was a phrase that was created, and no one is sure by whom, to supposedly denote a state of health. That state has been unable to be scientifically or medically defined or determined. It is used as a marketing gimmick.

Whole body metabolism. Same as "organism's metabolism." See "metabolism," above.

BIBLIOGRAPHY

American College of Sports Medicine. *Resource Manual for Guidelines for Exercise Testing and Prescription.* 2d ed. Baltimore: Williams & Wilkins, 1993.

———. *ACSM's Resource Manual for Guidelines for Exercise Testing and Prescription.* 3d ed. Baltimore: Williams & Wilkins, 1998.

Anderson, R., and A. Kozlovsky. "Chromium Intake, Absorption and Excretion of Subjects Consuming Self-Selected Diets." *American Journal of Clinical Nutrition* 41 (1985): 1177–83.

Anderson, S. A., and D. J. Raiten, eds. "Safety of Amino Acids Used as Dietary Supplements." *Federation of American Societies for Experimental Biology.* Bethesda, Md., 1992.

Arnheim, D. D., and W. E. Prentice. *Principles of Athletic Training.* 8th ed. St. Louis, Mo.: Mosby Year Book, 1993.

Arthritis Foundation. *Unproven Remedies Resource Manual.* Atlanta: Arthritis Foundation, 1991.

Barrett, S., and the editors of *Consumer Reports. Health Schemes, Scams, and Frauds.* Yonkers, N.Y.: Consumer Reports Books, 1990.

Barrett, S., and V. Herbert. *The Vitamin Pushers.* Amherst, N.Y.: Prometheus Books, 1994.

Barrett, S., et al. *Consumer Health: A Guide to Intelligent Decisions.* 7th ed. St. Louis: McGraw Hill, 2002.

Bender, A. *Health or Hoax: The Truth about Health Foods and Diets.* Amherst, N.Y.: Prometheus Books, 1986.

Bender, M., et al. "Trends in Prevalence and Magnitude of Vitamin and Mineral Usage and Correlation with Health Status." *Journal of the American Dietetics Association* 92 (1992): 1096–1101.

Bendich, A. "Safety Issues Regarding the Use of Vitamin Supplements." *Annals of New York Academy of Sciences* 669 (1992): 300–12.

Bennion, L. *Hypoglycemia: Fact or Fad?* New York: Crown Publishers, 1985.

Bennion, L. J., E. L. Berman, and J. M. Ferguson. *Straight Talk about Weight Control*. Yonkers, N.Y.: Consumer Reports Books, 1991.

Brody, J. E. "Experimental Evidence Is Lacking for Melatonin as Cure-all." *New York Times*, 27 September 1995, p. C9.

Butler, K. *A Consumer Guide to "Alternative" Medicine*. Amherst, N.Y.: Prometheus Books, 1992.

Butler, R., and J. A. Brody, eds. *Strategies to Delay Dysfunction in Later Life*. New York: Springer, 1995.

Byers, T. "Dietary Trends in the United States: Relevance to Cancer Prevention." *Cancer* 72 (1993): 1015–18.

Calle, Eugenia A., et al. "Body-Mass Index and Mortality in a Prospective Cohort of U.S. Adults." *New England Journal of Medicine* 341 (1999): 1097–1105.

Cleverley, W. O. *Essentials of Health Care Finance*. 4th ed. Gaithersburg, Md.: Aspen Publishers, 1997.

Cook-Fuller, C., and S. Barrett, eds. *Nutrition 93/94*. Guilford, Conn.: Dushkin Publishing, 1993.

Corti, M. C., et al. "HDL Cholesterol Predicts Coronary Heart Disease Mortality in Older Persons." *Journal of the American Medical Association* 274 (1995): 539.

Davidsson, L., et al. "The Effect of Individual Dietary Components on Manganese Absorption in Humans." *American Journal of Clinical Nutrition* 54 (1991): 1065–70.

Dean, W. *Biological Aging Measurement: Clinical Applications*. Los Angeles: Center for Bio-Gerontology, 1988.

Deutsch, R. *The New Nuts Among the Berries*. Palo Alto, Calif.: Bull Publishing Co., 1977.

Doyle, R. P. *The Medical Wars*. New York: William Morrow and Co., 1983.

DuPuy, N. A., and V. L. Mermel. *Focus on Nutrition*. St. Louis, Mo.: Mosby, 1995.

Durbin, R. J., et al. *Dietary Supplements*. Appropriations Subcommittee on Agriculture, Rural Development, Food and Drug Administration, and

Related Agencies, House Committee on Appropriations, 8 October 1993.

Dykstra, G. J., et al. *Dietary Supplements Task Force Report*. Rockville, Md.: Food and Drug Administration, 1992.

Eastwood, M. *Principles of Human Nutrition*. London: Chapman & Hall, 1997.

Fernandez-Brenares, F., E. Gine, and E. Cabre. "Factors Associated with Low Values of Biochemical Vitamin Parameters in Healthy Subjects." *International Journal of Vitamin Nutrition* 63 (1994): 68-74.

Finch, C. E. *Longevity, Senescence, and the Genome*. Chicago: University of Chicago Press, 1990.

Finch, C. E., and L. Hayflick, eds. *Handbook of the Biology of Aging*. New York: Van Norstrand, 1997.

Fishbein, M. *Fads and Quackery in Healing*. New York: Blue Ribbon Books, 1932.

Fleck, S. J., and W. J. Kraemer. *Designing Resistance Training Programs*. Champaign, Ill.: Human Kinetics Books, 1987.

Food and Drug Administration. "Food Labeling: General Requirements, Final and Proposed Rule." *Federal Register* 59, no. 2 (4 January 1994): 349-437.

Food and Drug Administration. "Unsubstantiated Claims and Documented Health Hazards in the Dietary Supplement Marketplace." Washington, D.C.: Food and Drug Administration, 1993.

Food and Nutrition Board, National Research Council. *Recommended Dietary Allowances*. 10th ed. Washington, D.C.: National Academy Press, 1989.

Fried, J. *Vitamin Politics*. Amherst, N.Y.: Prometheus Books, 1984.

Fries, J. F. "Aging, Natural Death and the Composition of Morbidity." *New England Journal of Medicine* (1980): 303-10.

Garland, D. "Ascorbic Acid and the Eye." *American Journal of Clinical Nutrition* 54 (1991): 1198S-1202S.

Garrison, R., Jr., and E. Somer. *The Nutrition Desk Reference*. New Canaan, Conn.: Keats Publishing, 1995.

Gavin, M., D. McCarthy, and P. Garry. "Evidence that Iron Stores Regulate Iron Absorption: A Setpoint Theory." *American Journal of Clinical Nutrition* 59 (1994): 1376-80.

Gershoff, S., and C. Whitney. *The Tufts University Guide to Total Nutrition*. New York: HarperCollins, 1992.

Ghigo, E., et al. "Arginine Potentiates the GHRH, but Not the

Pyridostigmine-Induced GH Secretion in Normal Short Children: Further Evidence for a Somatostatin Suppressing Effect of Arginine." *Clinical Endocrinology* 32 (1990): 763–67.

Haas, E. M. *Staying Healthy with Nutrition: The Complete Guide to Diet and Nutritional Medicine*. Berkeley, Calif.: Celestial Arts, 1992.

Hallberg, I., et al. "Calcium and Iron Absorption: Mechanisms of Action and Nutritional Importance." *European Journal of Clinical Nutrition* 46 (1992): 317–27.

Hay, L. E., and E. R. Wilson. *Accounting for Governmental and Nonprofit Entities*. 10th ed. Chicago: Irwin, 1995.

Hayflick, L. *How and Why We Age*. New York: Ballantine Books, 1994.

Heaney, R. "Calcium in the Prevention and Treatment of Osteoporosis." *Journal of Internal Medicine* 231 (1992): 169–80.

Herbert, V., and S. Barrett. *Vitamins and "Health" Foods: The Great American Hustle*. Philadelphia: George F. Strickley, 1981.

Herbert, V., and G. J. Subak-Sharpe, eds. *Total Nutrition: The Only Guide You'll Ever Need*. New York: St. Martin's Press, 1994.

Holliday, R. *Understanding Ageing*. Cambridge: Cambridge University Press, 1995.

Howley, E. T., and D. B. Franks. *Health Fitness Instructor's Handbook*. 3d ed. Champaign, Ill.: Human Kinetics, 1997.

Huber, P. *Galileo's Revenge: Junk Science in the Courtroom*. New York: Basic Books, 1991.

Jha, P., et al. "The Antioxidant Vitamins and Cardiovascular Disease: A Critical Review of Epidemiologic and Clinical Data." *Annals of Internal Medicine* 123 (1995): 860.

Jorgensen, J. O. L., et al. "Three Years of Growth Hormone Treatment in Growth Hormone-Deficient Adults: Near Normalization of Body Composition and Physical Performance." *European Journal of Endocrinology* 130 (1994): 224–28.

Katch, F. I., and W. D. McArdle. *Introduction to Nutrition, Exercise and Health*. 4th ed. Baltimore: Williams & Wilkins, 1993.

Katz, S., and H. Salem. "The Toxicology of Chromium with Respect to Its Chemical Speciation: A Review." *Journal of Applied Toxicology* 13 (1993): 217–24.

Katzel, L. I., et al. "Effects of Weight Loss vs. Aerobic Exercise Training on Risk Factors for Coronary Disease in Healthy, Obese, Middle-aged, and Older Men." *Journal of the American Medical Association* 272 (1995): 1915.

Keller, C.W. *Report of the Presiding Officer on Proposed Trade Regulation*

Rule Regarding Advertising and Labeling of Protein Supplements. Washington, D.C.: Federal Trade Commission, 15 June 1978.

Kleijinen, Knipschild. *British Medical Journal.* (1991). 302: 316–23

Kohrt, W. M., et al. "Effects of Gender, Age and Fitness Level on Response of VO_{2max} to Training in 60- to 70-year-olds." *Journal of Applied Physiology* 71 (1991): 2004.

Kronmal, H. M., et al. "Total Serum Cholesterol Levels and Mortality Risk as a Function of Age." *Archives of Internal Medicine* 153 (1993): 1065.

Lachance, P. "To Supplement or Not to Supplement: Is It a Question?" *Journal of the American College of Nutrition* 13 (1994): 113–15.

Langer, S. E., and J. F. Scheer. *Solved: The Riddle of Illness.* New Canaan, Conn.: Keats Publishing, 1984.

Lawton, W., et al. "Effect of Dietary Potassium on Blood Pressure, Renal Function, Muscle Sympathetic Nerve Activity, and Forearm Vascular Resistance and Flow in Normotensive and Borderline Hypertensive Humans." *Circulation* 81 (1990): 173–84.

Lenfant, C., and N. Ernst. "Daily Dietary Fat and Total Food Energy Intakes: NHANES III, Phase I, 1988–1991." *Journal of the American Medical Association* 271 (1994): 1309.

Leon, A. S., et al. "Physical Activity and 10.5 Year Mortality in the Multiple Risk Factor Intervention Trial (MRFIT)." *International Journal of Epidemiology* 20 (1991): 690.

Maddox, G. L., ed. *The Encyclopedia of Aging.* New York: Springer Publishing Company, 1995.

Manton, K. G., et al. "Longevity in the United States: Age and Sex-Specific Evidence on Life Span Limits from Mortality Patterns 1960-1990." *Journal of Gerontology: Biological Sciences* 51A:B362.

Marieb, E. N. *Human Anatomy and Physiology.* Redwood City, Calif.: Benjamin/Cummings Publishing Company, 1989.

Marshall, C. *Vitamins and Minerals: Help or Harm?* Philadelphia: J. B. Lippincott Co., 1985.

Martin, G. M. "Genetics of Human Disease, Longevity and Aging." In *Principles of Geriatric Medicine,* edited by R. Andres, E. L. Bierman, and W. R. Hazzard. New York: McGraw-Hill, 1985.

McAllister, M., K. Baghurst, and S. Record. "Financial Costs of Healthy Eating: A Comparison of Three Different Approaches." *Journal of Nutrition Education* 26 (1994): 131–39.

McArdle, W. D., F. I. Katch, and V. L. Katch. *Essentials of Exercise Physiology.* Baltimore: Williams & Wilkins, 1994.

Mertz, W. "Chromium: History of Nutritional Importance." *Biology of Trace Elements* 32 (1992): 3-8.

Meteseshe, J., et al. "Recovery of Dietary Iron and Zinc from the Proximal Intestine of Man: Studies of Different Meals and Supplements." *American Journal of Clinical Nutrition* 33 (1980): 1946.

Miller, R. A. "The Aging Immune System: Primer and Prospectus." *Science* 273 (1996): 70.

Mirkin, G. *Getting Thin*. Boston: Little Brown, 1983.

Naurath, H., et al. "Effects of Vitamin B_{12}, Folate, and Vitamin B_6 Supplements in Elderly People with Normal Serum Vitamin Levels." *Lancet* 346 (1995): 85.

Nelson, M. E. *Strong Women Stay Young*. New York: Bantam Books, 1997.

Newhouse, I., D. Clement, and C. Lai. "Effects of Iron Supplementation and Discontinuation on Serum Copper, Zinc, Calcium, and Magnesium Levels in Women." *Medicine and Science in Sport and Exercise* 25 (1993): 562-71.

Olshansky, S. J., et al. "In Search of Methuselah: Estimating the Upper Limits to Human Longevity." *Science* 250 (1990): 634.

Park, Y., I. Kim, and E. Yetley. "Characteristics of Vitamin and Mineral Supplement Products in the United States." *American Journal of Clinical Nutrition* 54 (1991): 750-59.

Payne, J. P. *Alternative Therapy*. British Medical Association, 1986.

Pennington, J., and B. Young. "Total Diet Study Nutritional Elements, 1982-1989." *Journal of the American Dietetics Association* 91 (1991): 179-83.

Pepper, C., et al. *Quackery: A $10 Billion Scandal*. Subcommittee on Health and Long-term Care of the Senate Select Committee on Aging, Washington, D.C., 31 May 1984.

Popov, I. M., and W. J. Goldway. "A Review of Properties and Clinical Effects of Ginseng." *American Journal of Chinese Medicine* 1, no. 2 (1973): 263-70.

Prince, R. L., et al. "Diet and the Prevention of Osteoporosis Fractures." *New England Journal of Medicine* 337 (1997): 701.

Raso, J. *Mystical Diets*. Amherst, N.Y.: Prometheus Books, 1993.

Reid, I. R., et al. "Effect of Calcium Supplement on Bone Loss in Postmenopausal Women." *New England Journal of Medicine* 328 (1993): 460.

Renner, J. *Health Smarts*. Kansas City, Mo.: Healthfacts Publishing, Inc., 1990.

Reynolds, R. "Vitamin Supplements: Current Controversies." *Journal of the American College of Nutrition* 13 (1994): 118-26.

Ricklefs, R. E., and C. E. Finch. *Aging: A Natural History.* New York: Scientific American Library, 1995.

Riggs, K. M., et al. "Relations of Vitamin B-12, Vitamin B-6, Folate and Homocysteine to Cognitive Performance in the Normative Aging Study." *American Journal of Clinical Nutrition* (1996): 63-306.

Rimm, E. B., et al. "Vitamin E Consumption and the Risk of Coronary Heart Disease in Men." *New England Journal of Medicine* 334 (1996): 1156.

————. "Vegetable, Fruit, and Cereal Fiber Intake and Risk of Coronary Heart Disease Among Men." *Journal of the American Medical Association* 257 (1996): 447.

Rosenfeld, I. *Modern Prevention: The New Medicine.* New York: Bantam Books, 1986.

Roth, W. V., et al. *Weight Reduction Products and Plans.* Permanent Subcommittee on Investigations, Senate Committee on Governmental Affairs, 14-15 May 1985.

Rowe, J. W., and R. L. Kahn. *Successful Aging.* New York: Pantheon Books, 1998.

Rudberg, M., et al. "Are Death and Disability in Old Age Preventable?" In *Facts and Research in Gerontology* 7, edited by J. L. Albarede, P. J. Garry, and D. Vallas, p. 791. New York: Springer (USA).

Rudman, D. "Growth Hormone, Body Composition and Aging." *Journal of American Geriatrics Society* 33 (1985): 800-807.

Sampson, W. *Skeptical Inquirer* (fall 1989).

Schaie, K. W., and S. L. Willis. "Can Decline in Adult Intellectual Function Be Reversed?" *Developmental Psychology* 22, no. 2 (1986): 223.

Scofield. *British Homeopathic Journal* 73 (1984): 161-226.

Seawell, L.V. *Hospital Financial Accounting: Theory and Practice.* 2d ed. Dubuque, Iowa: Kendall/Hunt Publishing Company, 1987.

Shils, M. E., et al. *Modern Nutrition in Health and Disease.* 9th ed. Baltimore: Williams & Wilkins, 1998.

Sifton, D. W., ed. *The PDR Pocket Guide to Prescription Drugs.* Rev. ed. New York: Pocket Books, 1997.

Siliprandi, N., and M. T. Ramacci. "Carnitine as a 'Drug' Affecting Lipid Metabolism." In *Coenzyme Q-10 and Clinical Aspects of Coenzyme 9,* edited by R. Fumagalli et al. Amsterdam: Biomedical Press, 1981.

Simopoulos, A., V. Herbert, and B. Jacobson. *Genetic Nutrition: Designing a Diet Based on Your Family Medical History.* New York: Macmillan, 1993.

Sizer, F. S., and E. N. Whitney. *Nutrition: Concepts and Controversies*. 6th ed. Eagan Publishing Co., 1994.

Spencer, H., L. Kramer, and D. Osis. "Effect of Calcium on Phosphorous Metabolism in Man." *American Journal of Clinical Nutrition* 40 (1984): 219-25.

Srikumar, T., et al. "Trace Element Status in Healthy Subjects Switching from a Mixed to a Lactovegetarian Diet for Twelve Months." *American Journal of Clinical Nutrition* 55 (1992): 885-90.

Stalker, D., and C. Glymour, eds. *Examining Holistic Medicine*. Amherst, N.Y.: Prometheus Books, 1985.

Stampfer, M. J., et al. "Postmenopausal Estrogen Therapy and Cardiovascular Disease." *New England Journal of Medicine* 325 (1991): 756.

Stare, F. J., and E. M. Phalen. *Panic in the Pantry*. Amherst, N.Y.: Prometheus Books, 1992.

Sticht, J. P., et al. "Weight Control and Exercise: Cardinal Features of Successful Preventive Gerontology" (editorial). *Journal of the American Medical Association* 274 (1995): 1964.

Subar, A., and G. Block. "Use of Vitamin and Mineral Supplements: Demographics and Amount of Nutrients Consumed." *American Journal of Epidemiology* 132 (1990): 1091-1101.

Suver, J. D., B. R. Neumann, and K. E. Boles. *Management Accounting for Healthcare Organizations*. 4th ed. Chicago: Precept Press, 1995.

Swain, David P., and Brian C. Leutholtz. *Metabolic Calculation Simplified*. Baltimore: Williams and Wilkins, 1997.

Thomas, C. L., ed. *Taber's Cyclopedic Medical Dictionary*. Philadelphia: F. A. Davis Company, 1993.

Tyler, V. *The Honest Herbal*. 4th ed. Binghamton, N.Y.: Haworth Press, 1999.

U.S. Departments of Agriculture and Health and Human Services. *Nutrition and Your Health: Dietary Guidelines for Americans*. (HG232). Washington, D.C.: U.S. Government Printing Office, 1985.

Ward, P. E., and R. D. Ward. *Encyclopedia of Weight Training*. Laguna Hills, Calif.: QPT Publications, 1991.

Waxman, H. A., et al. *Regulation of Dietary Supplements*. Subcommittee on Health and the Environment, House Committee on Energy and Commerce, 29 July 1993.

Wetle, T. "Living Longer, Aging Better." *Journal of the American Medical Association* 278 (1997): 1376.

Whiting, S. "Safety of Some Calcium Supplements Questioned." *Nutrition Review* 52 (1994): 95-97.

Willett, W. "Diet and Health: What Should We Eat?" *Science* 264 (1994): 532–37.

Williams, M. H. *The Ergogenics Edge*. Champaign, Ill.: Human Kinetics, 1998.

Winick, M., ed. *The Columbia Encyclopedia of Nutrition*. New York: G. P. Putnam's Sons, 1988.

Wyden, R., et al. *Deception and Fraud in the Diet Industry*. Subcommittee on Regulation, Business Opportunities, and Energy, House Subcommittee on Small Business, Washington, D.C., 26 and 27 March 1990.

Yetiv, J. *Popular Nutritional Practices: A Scientific Appraisal*. San Carlos, Calif.: Popular Medicine Press, 1986.

Young, J. H. *American Health Quackery*. Princeton, N.J.: Princeton University Press, 1992.

———. *The Medical Messiahs*. Princeton, N.J.: Princeton University Press, 1992.

INDEX

ABOUT THE AUTHOR

Dr. Larry Forness was born and raised in Denver, Colorado. He contracted nonpermanent paralysis from polio as a young child, which he overcame to excel in basketball, football, and baseball. He was educated in Catholic schools from kindergarten through his baccalaureate degree. He is also the child of alcoholic parents.

A specialist in sports medicine and exercise physiology, he did his undergraduate training at Notre Dame and took some of his advanced degrees and training from prestigious universities such as Duke University and UCLA. He also earned two law degrees (J.D. and I.L.M.).

Dr. Forness is the founder of the National Center for Sports Medicine and was its director for more than ten years. He was the producer and host of a one-hour, daily radio program called "Here's to Your Health," which was broadcast internationally over Radio Genesis. During the time Dr. Forness was serving as director of the National Center for Sports Medicine, he also created what is still believed to be the most comprehensive set of clinical tests, measurements, and examinations to determine a person's true age—called the biophysiological age. That test is called the L.I.F.E. TEST™, which stands for Longevity Indicator Functional Examination.

He is a member of the American College of Sports Medicine and holds its highest-level certification—Director of Health and Fitness—one of fewer than 250 health-care specialists in the world to hold that distinction. In addition, he was admitted to the American Academy of Anti-Aging Medicine, and was honored to write many of the questions for the first-ever board certification examinations on antiaging medicine. These examinations were given for the first time in December 1997. He is also a certified Healthcare Accountant and Financial Manager, awarded jointly by Indiana University's School of Business, the American Hospital Association, and the Healthcare Financial Management Association. He has authored many general health and fitness articles for newspapers and magazines.

Dr. Forness is also a member of the American Society for Human Genetics; the National Council for Reliable Health Information; the American Society of Law, Medicine & Ethics; and the Physicians and Scientists for the Responsible Application of Science and Technology.

He is a former United States Marine, is a licensed pilot (with Instrument Rating), and holds a First Degree Black Belt in TaeKwonDo. He is also an avid weightlifter and reads over three hundred books per year. He continues to perform classified consulting with various U.S. military entities in what the general public knows as "special operations" units. He has been personally involved in the health and fitness arena for over forty years.

Dr. Forness is currently a dean of a major health-care university in the southeastern United States, as well as serving as adjunct faculty at three other health-care universities.

The information in this book could save you money, frustration, embarrassment, and disappointment. It could even save your life!

Americans annually spend more than forty billion dollars—needlessly—on vitamins, minerals, herbal concoctions, ergogenic aids, fitness equipment and apparel, and alternative health-care treatments. In *Don't Get Duped!* Dr. Larry M. Forness provides the critical tools to help you evaluate the many health-care and fitness services and products available today. Using actual ads as examples, Forness presents the best ways to keep from ever being duped again by an industry that is rife with deception and ignorance, and also includes specific tips from industry "insiders."

The ultimate goal is to make you self-sufficient in appraising industry hype, and to give you the criteria to test real-world results against marketing claims. By judicious use of VIPs—Very Important Points—and concise checklists throughout the book, readers are given the most important facts in a readily usable form.

Topics covered include the real meaning of "scientifically proven"; methods for quantitatively analyzing such claims as "more energy" and "improved strength"; fad diets; fitness equipment; aging remedies; abuse of the labels "certified," "registered," and "licensed"; plus an extremely useful glossary.

Before you begin yet another weight-loss or fitness program or buy some new health-care product, you owe it to yourself to read what Dr. Forness has to say.

PROMETHEUS BOOKS
59 John Glenn Drive
Amherst, New York 14228-2197

www.prometheusbooks.com

Cover images © 2001 PhotoDisc, Inc.
Cover design by Grace M. Conti-Zilsberger

ISBN 1-57392-922-0

9 791573 929225

DR. LARRY M. FORNESS

is the founder of the National Center for Sports Medicine, and holds the highest professional certification—Director of Health Fitness—from the American College of Sports Medicine. He is also a member of Physicians and Scientists for Responsible Application of Science and Technology; the American Society for Human Genetics; the American Society for Law, Medicine, and Ethics; the Physicians' Committee for Responsible Medicine; and the National Council for Reliable Health Information.